Clinical
Management
of Shock

Clinical Management of Shock

David J. Kreis, Jr., M.D.

Chief, Trauma Section
Division of Emergency Surgical Services
Assistant Professor
Department of Surgery
University of Miami/Jackson Memorial Medical Center
Miami, Florida

Arthur E. Baue, M.D.

Donald Guthrie Professor of Surgery
Chairman, Department of Surgery
Yale University School of Medicine
and the Yale-New Haven Hospital
New Haven, Connecticut

University Park Press · Baltimore

University Park Press
International Publishers in Medicine and Allied Health
300 North Charles Street
Baltimore, Maryland 21201

Sponsoring editor: Marjorie Nelson
Production editor: Michael Treadway
Cover and text design by: Caliber Design Planning, Inc.

Typeset by: Waldman Graphics, Inc.
Manufactured in the United States of America by: Halliday Lithograph

Library of Congress Cataloging in Publication Data

Kreis, David J.
  Clinical management of shock.

  Includes index.
  1. Shock—Treatment. I. Baue, Arthur. II. Title.
[DNLM: 1. Shock—therapy. QZ 140 K92c]
RB150.S5K74   1984   616'.047   84-12018
ISBN 0-8391-2036-2

Contents

Preface

Coronary artery disease causes about 675,000 deaths per year. Most of these patients die from cardiogenic shock. In 1980 trauma claimed 164,000 lives in the United States and was the third leading cause of death. Furthermore, there are between 100,000 and 300,000 cases of Gram-negative bacteremia per year in the United States. About 20% of these patients develop septic shock, which carries a greater than 50% mortality risk.

It is clear that shock is a common clinical problem. It is important therefore for all physicians to understand the mechanisms of shock and the rationale for effective treatment.

This book starts with a review of the normal circulatory system and its control mechanisms. This background information is necessary so that the pathophysiologic alterations in shock will be understood. An introductory chapter on shock is next, followed by separate chapters on hemorrhagic (trauma), cardiogenic, septic, and neurogenic shock. Finally, a chapter on multiple organ system failure is included.

This book is intended for generalists. In particular, primary care physicians, emergency room physicians, internists, junior surgeons, house staff, and medical students should find it worthwhile reading. For the intended audience this book should bridge the gap between the pathogenesis of shock and its appropriate clinical management.

David J. Kreis, Jr., M.D.
Arthur E. Baue, M.D.

Acknowledgment

We wish to thank Ms. Robbie Butler, Ms. Cristina Martinez, and Ms. Helene Hoover for their expertise in the preparation of this monograph.

Notice

The author and the publisher have exercised great care to ensure that the drug dosages, formulas, and other information presented in this book are accurate and in accord with the professional standards in effect at the time of publication. Readers are, however, advised to always check the manufacturer's product information sheet that is packaged with the respective products to be fully informed of changes in recommended dosages, contraindications, and the like before prescribing or administering any drug.

The Normal Cardiovascular System and Its Control 1

Overview

This chapter focuses on the normal cardiovascular
system and its control mechanisms. The heart will
be discussed first. Consideration will be given to
the mechanisms of cardiac muscle contraction,
hemodynamics, myocardial energetics, and coronary blood flow. The vascular system will then be
discussed. This will include a description of the
different types of blood vessels, the determinants
of vascular control, and the mechanisms for control of blood flow. Cellular energetics, oxygen consumption and delivery, blood volume, and blood
pressure will be discussed. Finally, an integration
of the cardiac system and the vascular system will
be presented so that overall circulatory function,
including homeostatic mechanisms, may be understood. This is an important prerequisite in the understanding of the pathophysiology of shock.

Introduction

Shock is a common clinical problem, particularly
nowadays. With improvements in paramedic and
emergency medical services many acutely ill patients and victims of trauma are being successfully
treated at the scene and transported alive to the hospital. Trauma and heart disease are common causes
of shock. In 1980 trauma caused over 160,000 deaths
in the United States. It is the third leading cause of
death. Coronary heart disease causes 675,000 deaths
per year and is the leading cause of death.

Trauma and cardiac
disease are common
causes of shock.

It is important for all physicians to understand
the pathophysiology of shock and the rationale behind proper treatment. The major pathophysiologic
event in shock is diminished tissue perfusion. It is
this deficit in tissue perfusion and not hypotension
per se that is the essence of shock. Shock causes

3

cellular metabolic failure, organ dysfunction, and death. To adequately treat the patient in shock the inciting event must be controlled and tissue perfusion must be improved.

Shock results from circulatory failure.

Shock is the clinical manifestation of a failing circulation. The normal circulatory system should be viewed as a closed loop consisting of three interdependent components (Figure 1.1): 1) the heart (the pump), 2) the vessels (the conduits), and 3) the blood volume (the intravascular volume). Shock may be caused by a defect in any or all of these components. The target organ is the capillary bed, across which vital gases, metabolic nutrients, and waste products exchange.

One must have knowledge of the normal circulation and its control in order to understand the homeostatic mechanisms of the cardiovascular system during shock. This involves an integration of the cardiac system with the vascular system.

▇ The Heart

Cardiac muscle is composed of myocardial cells or fibers about 40–100 μm (micrometers) long and 10–20 μm in diameter (Figure 1.2). These cells are composed of parallel arrangements of myofibrils, which are in turn made up of numerous serially repeating units called sarcomeres. Sarcomeres are the basic contractile units of muscle and are composed of the contractile proteins actin and myosin. Sarcomeres occupy about 50% of the mass of the cardiac muscle cell and about 90% of the mass of the skeletal muscle cell. Mitochondria, the intracellular organelles responsible for generating the energy substrate required for protein contraction, occupy spaces between the myofibrils and account for 20–30% of the cardiac cell mass.

Sarcomeres are the basic contractile units of the myocardial cell.

Myosin is composed of light and heavy meromyosin. The light meromyosin forms the linear backbone of the total myosin protein molecule, whereas the heavy meromyosin protrudes away from the light meromyosin. The globular head of heavy meromyosin forms cross-links or bridges with actin

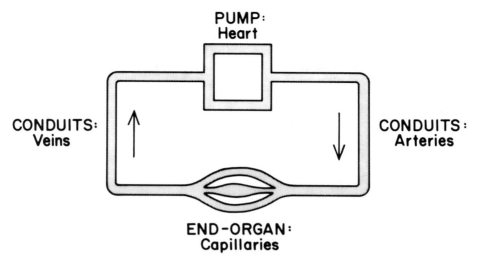

FIGURE 1.1 The circulatory system can be viewed as a closed loop made up of three parts: 1) the heart (the pump), 2) the blood vessels (the conduits), and 3) the blood volume (the intravascular volume).

during muscle contraction. Two additional proteins, tropomyosin and troponin, are associated with actin and are necessary for normal contraction. Troponin normally inhibits the interaction of actin and myosin.

Depolarization of the muscle cell membrane initiates the contraction process. When the muscle cell membrane is depolarized, calcium is released by the sarcoplasmic reticulum. The sarcoplasmic reticulum is a membranous tubular network which intimately surrounds the myofibrils. The calcium released by this system during depolarization binds to the troponin protein and removes troponin's inhibitory function. Actin and myosin can then form cross-bridges. These cross-bridges can be viewed as hinges, so that the actin molecule can slide on the myosin molecule within the sarcomere unit. The length of the sarcomere diminishes and the myocardial cell contracts. The energy necessary for this process comes from the hydrolysis of adenosine triphosphate (ATP) by the enzyme adenosine triphosphatase (ATPase), which is associated with the myosin molecule.

The actin and myosin proteins overlap each

The energy necessary for muscle contraction comes from ATP.

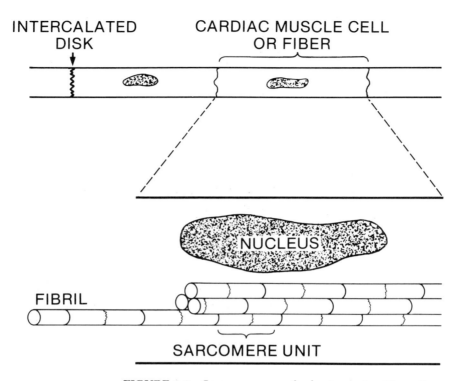

INTERCALATED
DISK

CARDIAC MUSCLE CELL
OR FIBER

NUCLEUS

FIBRIL

SARCOMERE UNIT

FIGURE 1.2   Sarcomeres are the basic contractile units
of the myocardial cell. They occupy about 50% of the
mass of the cardiac muscle cell. Adapted from
Braunwald E, Ross J Jr, Sonnenblick EH. Mechanisms of
Contraction of the Normal and Failing Heart. Little,
Brown, Boston, 1976, p 3.

Sarcomere length is
related to ventricular
volume and pressure.

other within the sarcomere units so that the number
of potential coupling sites between the two proteins
varies with sarcomere length. The optimal sarcomere
length required for maximal muscle tension development is 2.2 μm. In the heart, sarcomere length is
related to ventricular volume and pressure. When
the left ventricle is empty of blood volume, the sarcomere length is about 1.9 μm. By steadily increasing left ventricular filling volume and, subsequently,
left ventricular filling pressure, the sarcomere length
can be stretched so that the maximal number of potential coupling sites between the actin and myosin
molecules is attained. The ideal sarcomere length of
2.2 μm is attained when the left ventricular diastolic

pressure reaches 12–15 mm Hg and the right ventricular diastolic pressure reaches 8–10 mm Hg.

Cardiac Hemodynamics

The primary function of the heart is to effect adequate perfusion of the capillaries. The physiologic expression of this effected blood flow is called the cardiac output. It is the quantity of blood moved per minute by the heart from the venous system to the arterial system. In the average supine adult it measures about 5.6 liters/min or 3.0 ± 0.5 liters/min/m^2 of body surface area (cardiac index). Cardiac output can vary normally from a value during standing position that is 25% below the output during supine position, up to a value during severe exercise that is 8 times the normal resting supine value.

Cardiac output (CO) equals the product of heart rate (HR) times stroke volume (SV):

$$CO = HR \times SV$$

Stroke volume is the volume of blood ejected by the heart per cardiac contraction. It is measured by subtracting the volume of blood in the ventricle at the end of systole from the volume of blood in the ventricle at the end of diastole. In the average supine resting adult stroke volume measures about 70 ml or 40 ± 7 ml/m^2 of body surface area (stroke index). The fraction of ventricular end-diastolic blood volume ejected per contraction, called the ejection fraction, is at least 50% in the normal resting adult.

If the stroke volume is held constant, then cardiac output varies as a linear function of heart rate. Although the sinoatrial node receives sympathetic and parasympathetic innervation via the cardiac and vagus nerves, respectively, under usual physiologic conditions heart rate is determined by the intrinsic rhythmicity of the sinoatrial node pacemaker cells. This intrinsic regulation is a function of the metabolic rate of the sinoatrial node itself.

Varying the heart rate per se usually does not alter cardiac output significantly due to concomitant changes in stroke volume. Those conditions that usually cause a sinus tachycardia (fear, exercise, etc.) also usually cause an activation of the entire cardio-

Cardiac output = 5.6 liters/min
Cardiac index = 3.0 ± 0.5 liters/min/m^2

Cardiac output equals stroke volume times heart rate:
$CO = HR \times SV$

Stroke volume = 70 ml
Stroke index = 40 ± 7 ml/m^2

Cardiac output is regulated mainly by stroke volume. Stroke volume depends on cardiac preload, afterload, and contractility.

vascular system such that stroke volume is increased as well.

The regulation of cardiac output and cardiac performance is, therefore, mainly achieved via regulation of stroke volume. The magnitude of stroke volume is determined by the degree of myocardial cell shortening during contraction. This is controlled by three factors: 1) the preload, 2) the afterload, and 3) the contractile state or contractility of the myocardium.

Preload

Preload is the amount of stretch put on the cardiac muscle cell prior to contraction. This stretch will determine the degree of shortening of the cardiac muscle during contraction and the strength of muscle contraction. Increasing the preload up to the optimal sarcomere length of 2.2 μm will increase the

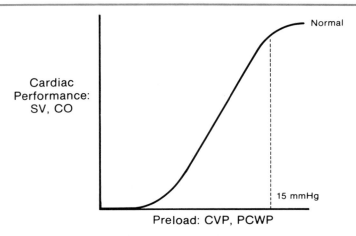

FIGURE 1.3 The ventricular function curve is a graphic way to portray cardiac performance as a function of preload. Preload and cardiac performance reach a plateau stage at a PCWP of 15 mm Hg. Numerous factors can affect preload, including blood volume, body position, intrathoracic and intrapericardial pressure, venous tone, atrial contraction, and the pumping action of skeletal muscle. Reprinted with permission from Kreis DJ Jr. Shock (Part I): Pathophysiology. Curr Rev Respir Ther 6:60, 1983.

stroke volume. Beyond this level of stretch the potential coupling sites between actin and myosin decrease so that there is less shortening and less contraction strength. The relationship between preload (measured as diastolic muscle length) and strength of contraction (measured as systolic muscle tension) is known as the Frank-Starling relationship or Starling's law of the heart.

The Frank-Starling relationship relates diastolic length to systolic tension.

Preload is usually expressed as the pressure in the ventricle at the end of diastole, or the end-diastolic filling pressure. This pressure is a direct function of the volume of blood in the ventricle at the end of diastole, or the end-diastolic filling volume. Preload is thus proportional to the end-diastolic filling volume. Normally, an increase in end-diastolic filling volume is accompanied by an increase in end-diastolic filling pressure. Since the average resting stroke volume in the supine adult is about 70 ml, about 70 ml of venous blood must be delivered to the heart prior to each contraction. If cardiac output is to be maintained at a specific level, then the amount of venous return must equal the amount of stroke volume per contraction.

To maintain cardiac output, venous return must equal the amount of stroke volume per contraction.

Various factors affect the preload. These include body position, blood volume, intrathoracic and intrapericardial pressure, venous tone, pumping action of skeletal muscle, and the efficiency of atrial contraction. As examples, in pericardial tamponade the intrapericardial pressure increases so that the heart cannot distend in order to receive venous return. In tension pneumothorax the elevated positive intrathoracic pressure compresses the great veins of the thorax and inhibits ventricular filling. In atrial fibrillation the contribution of the atria to the ventricular filling is lost.

Factors that influence preload

The Frank-Starling relationship is best expressed as a ventricular function curve relating preload to cardiac performance (Figure 1.3). Clinically, preload of the right ventricle is obtained by measuring the right atrial pressure or the central venous pressure (CVP). The CVP is the pressure measured within the superior vena cava and is normally less than 10 cm H_2O. The preload of the left ventricle, or the left ventricular end-diastolic pressure (LVEDP), is obtained by measuring the mean pulmonary capillary wedge pressure (PCWP) or the pulmonary artery diastolic pressure (PADP) using a Swan-Ganz

The ventricular function curve relates preload to cardiac performance.

Normal CVP is below 10 cm H_2O.

balloon flotation catheter. The mean PCWP is the mean pressure within a small distal branch of one of the pulmonary arteries. It reflects directly the mean pressure within the pulmonary capillary and pulmonary venous systems. It measures 6–12 mm Hg normally. The PADP is the pressure within the pulmonary artery during diastole. It usually is only slightly higher than the mean PCWP, by 1–3 mm Hg. In most cases the PADP can be used to approximate the PCWP. There are some important exceptions, however, as in pulmonary hypertension. A detailed discussion of CVP, PCWP, and PADP and their clinical applications is found in the section on "Patient Monitoring" in Chapter 2. Cardiac performance is measured as either cardiac output or cardiac index, stroke volume or stroke index, or stroke work, which is the product of stroke volume and mean aortic pressure.

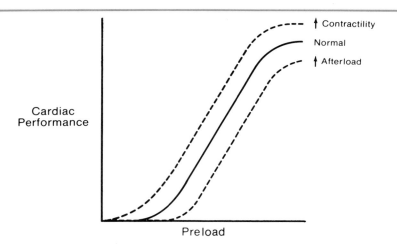

FIGURE 1.4   Changes in afterload and myocardial contractility affect the position of the ventricular function curve. An increase in afterload causes the function curve to shift downward and to the right, so that for each preload there is a decrease in cardiac performance. An increase in myocardial contractility has the opposite effect. Several factors influence the inotropic state of the heart, including autonomic nervous system influences, endogenous catecholamines, and inotropic drugs. Reprinted with permission from Kreis DJ Jr. Shock (Part I): Pathophysiology. Curr Rev Respir Ther 6:60, 1983.

From the ventricular function curve one sees that the initial linear relationship between preload and cardiac performance reaches a plateau stage starting at about 10 mm Hg for LVEDP. Left ventricular filling pressures greater than 15–18 mm Hg do not significantly increase cardiac performance via the Frank-Starling mechanism.

Left ventricular filling pressures greater than 15–18 mm Hg do not increase cardiac output via the Frank-Starling mechanism.

Afterload

The second factor that regulates stroke volume is the afterload, which is the resistance to forward blood flow caused by aortic pressure and total peripheral vascular resistance. This resistance force is equivalent to the tension that the heart must develop during contraction to cause forward blood flow. In general, a decrease in cardiac afterload causes an increase in stroke volume and cardiac output, whereas an increase in cardiac afterload has the opposite effect. Changes in the afterload can, therefore, affect the position of the ventricular function curve (Figure 1.4). Decreases in the afterload are associated with a leftward shift in the ventricular function curve, which signifies improved cardiac performance.

Afterload is resistance to forward blood flow.

The heart is capable of adapting to increases in afterload in order to maintain normal cardiac output. For example, if the aortic pressure is increased acutely, the force of ventricular contraction that was governed by the previous preload will not be enough to effect the same stroke volume. The stroke volume will be less and the end-diastolic volume will increase. To this residual volume will be added another preload volume during the subsequent diastole. This results in a new, larger preload, and the next systole will show an increased stroke volume due to the increased preload (via the Frank-Starling mechanism). The heart can compensate for elevations in cardiac afterload in this manner but at the expense of increasing ventricular size.

Contractility

The third factor controlling stroke volume is the contractility of the myocardium (inotropy). Contractility

Contractility is related to the force of contraction and velocity of shortening.

is related to the force of contraction and the velocity of shortening during contraction. Independent of preload and afterload, changes in myocardial contractility cause changes in myocardial performance. There exists a unique velocity of shortening for each level of preload and afterload. Classically, contractility is defined by the maximum velocity of shortening (or V_{max}) when afterload is zero. Various indexes of contractility besides V_{max} have been defined. These include measurements of ventricular volume, intraventricular pressure, relationships between ventricular wall tension and fiber length, the rate of pressure change (or dp/dt), and wall thickness.

Contractility affects the position of the ventricular function curve.

Changes in myocardial contractility are difficult to detect directly using the parameters listed above. Usually, changes in the contractile state of the myocardium are expressed by means of the ventricular function curve (Figure 1.4). Increases in contractility cause a leftward shift in the function curve. Decreases in contractility have the opposite effect. Performance can vary independently of the loading conditions placed on the heart. The ability to alter performance without altering the initial myocardial length (preload) is called homeometric regulation. The contractile state of the myocardium is controlled mainly by the sympathetic division of the autonomic nervous system. Increased sympathetic activity will cause a leftward shift in the ventricular function curve and thereby improve cardiac performance. Adrenal medullary hormones and inotropic drugs have the same effect.

Myocardial Energetics

The heart at rest normally uses free fatty acids as its major fuel source, but glucose, lactate, acetate, and acetoacetate can also be metabolized to generate acetyl-CoA and ultimately carbon dioxide and water. Energy production is essential for normal cellular function. Under aerobic conditions the combustion of 1 mole of glucose yields 38 moles of ATP, which is the energy substrate needed for contraction. This is accomplished via the glycolytic process, the Krebs cycle, and the electron-transport chain mechanism. This is discussed in further detail in Chapter 2 under "Cellular Energetics."

Coronary Blood Flow

The basal oxygen need of the myocardium without regard for the contraction process is about 2 ml O_2/min/100 g. This represents about 20% of the total oxygen needed by the normal beating heart at rest, which is about 10 ml O_2/min/100 g. The electrical activity of the heart requires 0.04 ml O_2/min/100 g. Myocardial oxygen consumption is directly proportional to coronary blood flow. Most of coronary blood flow (70%) occurs during diastole. Normal coronary flow at rest is about 5% of the cardiac output, or 250 ml/min, or 80 ml/min/100 g. The heart must extract about 65–70% of the oxygen delivered to it at normal coronary flow rates in order to support its basal oxygen requirement. This normal resting rate of oxygen extraction is about the maximal rate achieved by skeletal muscle during severe exercise. Thus, the heart cannot increase the efficiency of its oxygen extraction. Oxygen delivery to the heart can only be improved by increasing the coronary flow. For example, during maximum exercise, the heart needs up to 50 ml O_2/min/100 g, which would require a coronary blood flow of 350–400 ml/min/100 g.

Coronary blood flow is directly proportional to aortic pressure and inversely proportional to coronary vascular resistance. In the normal heart, coronary flow is mainly related to changes in coronary vascular resistance. Furthermore, coronary blood flow is normally autoregulated so that between aortic pressures of 60 and 120 mm Hg coronary blood flow remains constant. Autoregulation of blood flow is the process whereby blood flow is maintained constant despite fluctuations in blood pressure.

Other factors are involved in determining coronary vascular resistance. Mechanical factors are important. When the heart contracts, coronary flow is decreased due to the increased resistance caused by the compression of intramyocardial vessels. This compressive force accounts for 25% of the coronary vascular resistance at rest. During tachycardia, however, this effect may contribute up to 50% of the coronary vascular resistance because of the increased percentage of time spent in systole. Metabolic factors are also involved in controlling coronary vascular resistance. A decreased partial pressure of oxygen (PO_2) is a more potent stimulus for coro-

Myocardial O_2 consumption is directly proportional to myocardial blood flow. The myocardium extracts 65–70% of the O_2 delivered to it.

Coronary blood flow is normally autoregulated.

nary vasodilatation than is an increased partial pressure of carbon dioxide (PCO_2). Other factors include blood pH, concentration of adenine nucleotides, and perhaps various prostaglandin hormones. Sympathetic nervous system stimulation usually causes enhanced coronary blood flow mostly by improving the inotropic state of the myocardium rather than by causing coronary vasodilation.

The Vascular System

There are five main types of blood vessels.

There are five types of blood vessels: 1) large elastic arteries, 2) resistance vessels (arterioles, precapillary sphincters), 3) exchange vessels (capillaries, some venules), 4) capacitance vessels (veins), and 5) shunt vessels (arteriovenous [A-V] anastomoses).

The Arterial System

The aorta and large arteries have more collagen and less smooth muscle in their walls than do small arteries. The elastic elements within the larger arterial walls allow them to be stretched during systolic ejection to accommodate the stroke volume. These vessels thereby store some of the energy exerted during cardiac contraction (windkessel vessels). This phenomenon converts pulsatile systolic ejection into constant peripheral flow. Pulsatile flow ends at the arterioles. Blood flow through the capillaries and small venules is constant. About 20% of the total blood volume is contained within the arterial system at any one time.

The Microcirculation

The microcirculation comprises those vessels less than 100 μm in diameter. These include the terminal arterioles, the metarterioles, the capillaries, the A-V shunt channels, and the postcapillary venules (Figure 1.5).

The arteriole system is a resistance system. Most of the systolic pressure drop occurs across the arte-

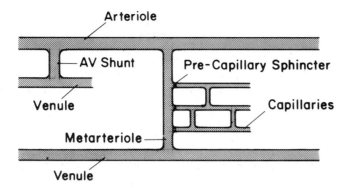

5 Types of Blood Vessels:

   1. Large Elastic Arteries

   2. Resistance Vessels − Arterioles, Sphincters

   3. Exchange Vessels − Capillaries, Venules

   4. Capacitance Vessels − Veins

   5. Shunt Vessels − AV Anastomoses

FIGURE 1.5 There are five types of blood vessels. The microcirculation includes those vessels less than 100 μm in diameter. Reprinted with permission from Zweifach BW, Functional Behavior of the Microcirculation. Charles C Thomas, Springfield IL, 1961, p 10.

rioles. In general, the arterioles cause 80% of the total peripheral vascular resistance, whereas the venules cause 20%. The metarteriole is a high-resistance, direct channel between arteriole and venule. In general the capillaries branch off of these metarterioles. Capillary flow is governed by the precapillary sphincter located at the junction of the capillary with the metarteriole. The precapillary sphincter is the final neuromuscular control point of the capillary blood flow. The arterioles, metarterioles, and precapillary sphincters are all under sympathetic nervous control. Their degree of vasoconstriction depends also on endogenous catecholamines and local metabolites. Temperature, pH, PO_2, and PCO_2 are factors that can affect the tone of the precapillary sphincters.

    In skin, intestine, and possibly kidney, there exist A-V shunt anastomoses to shunt blood flow quickly from artery to vein as needed. They are larger in diameter but shorter than metarterioles, and capillaries do not branch off of them. An example of their importance is that they enable the skin to dissipate heat rapidly.

About 5% of the total blood volume is contained within capillaries. Capillaries average about 5–20 μm in diameter and 0.4–0.7 mm in length. Transit time through a capillary is about 0.7 seconds.

Capillary blood flow is locally regulated by vasomotion.

Capillary blood flow is regulated at the local level by capillary vasomotion whereby the precapillary sphincters periodically contract and relax in response to the effects of local metabolites.

Capillary exchange via Starling's hypothesis

Capillary exchange refers to the mechanism by which substances exchange between the capillary and the interstitial space between cells. Capillary exchange of fluid occurs mainly by diffusion in accordance with Starling's hypothesis for capillary exchange. This hypothesis states that capillary exchange is determined not only by the difference in hydrostatic pressure between capillary and tissue (the filtration pressure) but also by the difference in colloid osmotic pressure between plasma and tissue. The colloid osmotic pressure is the osmotic pressure due to plasma proteins or colloids. The plasma colloid osmotic pressure tends to keep fluid within the vascular system, whereas the filtration pressure tends to push fluid out of the vascular system.

In the pulmonary circulation the pressures are much lower, and thus exchange favors reabsorption away from the interstitial space. In the renal circulation, on the other hand, the high glomerular capillary pressure favors production of capillary filtrate. The venous end of the capillary is 60% more permeable in general than the arterial end. Venules may also be involved in exchange processes.

The Venous System

The veins act as conduits and reservoirs.

The venous system has two major purposes: 1) to act as a conduit to return unoxygenated blood to the heart and 2) to act as a low-pressure reservoir for blood storage. About 75% of the total blood volume is contained within the veins at any one time. They are capacitance vessels. The venous capacitance is about 20 times greater than the arterial capacitance. For example, if the venous pressure increases by 1

Venous capacitance is 20 times greater than arterial capacitance.

mm Hg, then 20 times more blood volume could be stored in the venous side than could be stored in the arterial side for the same pressure increase.

Control of the Vascular System

Various factors influence vascular tone and ultimately capillary blood flow. The functional result of vascular control is the appropriate distribution of flow necessary for tissue metabolic needs. In general, vascular smooth muscle tone is controlled by four factors: 1) intrinsic mechanisms, 2) the autonomic nervous system, 3) endogenous catecholamines and vasoactive hormones, and 4) local metabolic factors.

Vascular smooth muscle tone is controlled by four factors.

The precapillary sphincters, the arterioles, and some postcapillary venules have single-unit smooth muscle cells that function as pacemaker cells due to spontaneous membrane depolarization. These smooth muscle pacemaker cells regulate capillary blood flow. The rate of pacemaker cell activity (or vasomotor activity) is related to the pressure within the microcirculation (the Bayliss hypothesis). Passively stretching these cells increases their discharge rate and thereby increases vascular tone. Feedback mechanisms exist to regulate the intrinsic activity of these pacemaker cells. In other words, the continuous stretch caused by blood pressure causes positive feedback (increased vascular tone), whereas the cumulative effects of local tissue metabolites causes negative feedback (decreased vascular tone).

Precapillary sphincters act as gateways controlling capillary flow.

Vascular tone is mainly regulated by the autonomic nervous system, in particular the sympathetic adrenergic vasoconstrictor fibers, which receive input from the cardiovascular center of the medulla. Neural input from higher cortical areas also may regulate this system. It is interesting to note that, although unmyelinated sympathetic and parasympathetic fibers travel with the arterioles, to date there is no proof that these nerve fibers actually make synaptic contact with either vascular smooth muscle cells, endothelial cells, or pericytes. These nerve fibers do, however, release a neurotransmitter (norepinephrine) that regulates vascular tone.

The autonomic nervous system sets the vascular tone.

Two additional types of autonomic nervous system fibers influence vascular tone. The sympathetic cholinergic vasodilating fibers are limited mainly to the arterioles of skeletal muscle. These fibers regulate the vasodilation that occurs in muscle prior to exercise, with emotional upset, and with any fight-or-flight reaction. The parasympathetic cholinergic vasodilating fibers play a small role in the overall control of vascular tone but are known to cause vasodilation of the vessels of the pia mater and external genitalia.

There are different types of vascular receptors.

Endogenous catecholamines also regulate vascular tone. They do so by binding to protein receptors located in vessel walls. There are several types of vascular receptors. These include: 1) α-adrenergic receptors (causing vasoconstriction) located in skin, intestine, muscle, kidney, and mucosal membranes; 2) β_1-adrenergic receptors (causing increased cardiac inotropic and chronotropic properties) located in cardiac muscle and β_2-adrenergic receptors (causing vasodilation) located in skeletal muscle and in pulmonary and mesenteric vascular beds; and 3) dopaminergic receptors (causing vasodilation) located in renal and mesenteric vascular beds. In addition to the endogenous catecholamines (epinephrine, norepinephrine, dopamine), various vasoactive amines (histamine, serotonin), glucocorticoids, estrogens, and even adenine nucleotides may play some role in regulating vascular tone.

Metabolic factors that affect vascular tone

Finally, metabolic factors can directly influence vascular tone. In most tissues a decrease in PO_2 or an increase in PCO_2 will cause vasodilation and increase local blood flow. An exception to this generalization is found in the pulmonary circulation. To maintain a balanced ventilation-to-perfusion ratio in the lung, a decrease in PO_2 will cause pulmonary vasoconstriction.

Tissue Blood Flow

The amount of blood flow to various tissues depends on the metabolic needs of those tissues. If blood flow to a particular tissue changes, this change must be accompanied by either a reciprocal change in flow to other tissues or a change in cardiac output. Redistribution of flow plays some role in the body's response to different stressful stimuli (exercise, blood loss, etc.). Most changes in blood flow, however, are accompanied by changes in cardiac output. The distribution of the cardiac output to the peripheral tissues varies from tissue to tissue. Coronary blood flow and its regulation have been discussed earlier.

Most changes in blood flow are accompanied by changes in cardiac output.

Brain

Cerebral blood flow is regulated mainly by PO_2, PCO_2, and local metabolites. Hypercarbia (high PCO_2) is a much more potent stimulus for cerebral vasodilation than is hypoxia (low PO_2). For example, an acute increase in PCO_2 to 52 mm Hg will raise cerebral blood flow by 70%. A decrease in PCO_2 of similar magnitude will not cause the same degree of reciprocal change in cerebral blood flow. Hypoxia does not cause cerebral vasodilation until the PO_2 drops below 50 mm Hg. Controversy still exists as to whether or not the change in cerebral blood flow found in hypercarbic states is secondary to the PCO_2 directly or to changes in pH.

The cerebral vessels are richly innervated by sympathetic fibers. However, changes in the tone of these fibers play little role in the regulation of cerebral blood flow. Indeed, cerebral blood flow, like coronary and renal blood flow, is autoregulated over a wide range of blood pressures. Cerebral blood flow does not decrease until the blood pressure drops below 70 mm Hg. Intracranial pressure above 30 mm Hg will decrease cerebral blood flow. Cerebral blood flow is about 12% of the cardiac output, or 50 ml/min/100 g. This corresponds to an oxygen consumption of 3 ml O_2/min/100 g. The clinical symptoms of cerebral ischemia do not occur until flow has been reduced to 60% of normal.

Cerebral blood flow is autoregulated.

Kidney

The kidneys receive about 20% of the cardiac output. Most renal blood flow occurs in the renal cortex rather than in the renal medulla (1–2%). The renal cortex is capable of autoregulating renal blood flow over a wide range of blood pressures, from 90 mm Hg to

Renal blood flow is autoregulated.

Glomerular filtration rate decreases at blood pressures less than 90 mm Hg.

200 mm Hg. Renal blood flow and glomerular filtration rate decrease at blood pressures below 90 mm Hg. Urine formation ceases at a blood pressure of about 50 mm Hg. Renal oxygen consumption is about 18 ml/min or 9 ml/min/100 g for renal cortex and 0.4 ml/min/100 g for inner medulla.

Sympathetic innervation of the renal vessels has some control over the magnitude of renal vasoconstriction. Severe hypoxia causes renal vasoconstriction. This effect is mediated via the carotid and aortic arch chemoreceptors. Severe hypercarbia can also cause renal vasoconstriction. Bacterial pyrogens can cause renal vasodilation. This effect is independent of any associated febrile reaction.

Lung

The pulmonary circulation is a low-resistance system.

The pulmonary circulation is a low-resistance system. Pulmonary blood flow can increase greatly with little change in driving pressure. For example, exercise will cause pulmonary blood flow to increase severalfold due to increased cardiac output, whereas there will be little change in pulmonary arterial pressure. Because of its low resistance the pulmonary circulation can act as a blood reservoir. In a normal adult assumption of the supine position will increase the pulmonary blood volume by about 400 ml and will cause a decrease in vital capacity. In heart failure these changes may cause clinical orthopnea.

Splanchnic Bed, Skeletal Muscle, and Skin

The splanchnic circulation includes three parts: 1) the splanchnic bed, 2) the hepatic bed, and 3) the splenic bed. All three areas are under sympathetic nervous system control via the splanchnic nerves. These nerves can cause vasoconstriction. There is no evidence at present that they carry vasodilator fibers.

Splanchnic blood flow is 25% of the cardiac output at rest.

Splanchnic blood flow is 1500 ml/min or about 25% of the normal resting cardiac output. The liver receives about 75% of its blood flow via the portal vein and about 25% via the hepatic artery. Like the splanchnic arteries, the portal vein is innervated by sympathetic vasoconstrictor fibers.

At rest, blood flow to skeletal muscle is about 850 ml/min or 15% of the cardiac output. This corresponds to an oxygen consumption of about 0.2 ml/min/100 g.

Skeletal muscle blood flow is 15% of the cardiac output at rest.

The cutaneous circulation is under sympathetic adrenergic vasoconstrictor control. The skin does not contain vasodilator fibers. Normal skin blood flow is about 460 ml/mm or 8% of the cardiac output. This corresponds to an oxygen consumption of 0.3 ml/min/100 g. Elevated body temperature dilates skin vessels (less vasoconstriction). Local heat has the same effect. Exercise causes cutaneous vasodilation secondary to elevated body temperature, despite increased sympathetic activity.

▓▓▓ Blood Volume

The normal adult blood volume varies between 4 and 4.5 liters (67 ml/kg) for the female and between 5 and 5.5 liters (75 ml/kg) for the male. Both short- and long-term mechanisms exist for the regulation of blood volume.

Short- and long-term mechanisms exist to regulate blood volume.

One short-term mechanism for maintaining the blood volume is via Starling's law of capillary exchange. For example, one of the body's responses to an acute decrease in blood volume, say from hemorrhage, is arteriolar vasoconstriction. This causes a decrease in capillary pressure and thus filtration pressure. This will result in a net transfer of fluid from the interstitial space into the intravascular space. An increase in plasma (blood) volume will result.

Blood volume regulation via capillary exchange

Normal blood volume
      Female: 4.0–4.5 liters or 67 ml/kg
      Male: 5.0–5.5 liters or 75 ml/kg
Normal control of blood volume
      Plasma refill
      ADH
      Aldosterone
      Erythropoietin

Blood volume regula-
tion via red blood cell
production

This process is called plasma refill, and the details of it are discussed in Chapter 2 under the heading "Volume Adjustments."

Long-term mechanisms include the regulation of red blood cell production as well as those factors that cause an increase in plasma volume. The precise control mechanism for red blood cell production is unknown. Hypoxia, however, can cause an increase in red blood cell production due to its stimulating effect on erythropoietin release from the kidney. Although the mechanism of plasma protein control is unknown, the total amount of plasma protein is the most important determinant of plasma volume.

Blood volume regula-
tion via water and salt
conservation

Plasma volume is controlled also by the amount of sodium and total body water present. Antidiuretic hormone (ADH) and aldosterone both play a vital role in water and sodium homeostasis. In hypovolemic states they are secreted in order to conserve water and sodium. The end result of their action is reflected in a diminished urine output and a decrease in the amount of sodium excreted in the urine.

ADH is released from the posterior pituitary and controls water reabsorption in the distal convoluted tubules and collecting tubules of the kidney. It is released in response to: 1) osmoreceptors of the supraoptic nucleus of the hypothalamus and 2) changes in extracellular fluid volume via stretch receptors located in both cardiac atria. These atrial receptors have neural connections with the posterior pituitary.

Aldosterone is secreted by the zona glomerulosa of the adrenal cortex. It controls sodium and water reabsorption at the distal tubule of the nephron. This causes isotonic volume expansion. Aldosterone is released 1) in response to adrenocorticotropic hormone (ACTH) released from the anterior pituitary and 2) via the renin-angiotensin system. A decrease in pulse pressure or mean blood pressure causes the renal juxtaglomerular cells to secrete renin. Renin enzymatically converts renin substrate (or angiotensinogen) into angiotensin I. This decapeptide is converted to the octapeptic angiotensin II in the pulmonary circulation. Angiotensin II both is vasoactive (causing vasoconstriction) and acts as a stimulus for aldosterone secretion. Furthermore, angiotensin II acts as a negative feedback control inhibiting further renin production.

Blood Pressure

Blood pressure is the driving force behind blood flow. It is directly proportional to the product of blood flow and resistance to blood flow as follows:

blood pressure (BP) = cardiac output (CO) × total peripheral resistance (TPR)
= heart rate (HR) × stroke volume (SV) × total peripheral resistance (TPR)

$$BP = CO \times TPR$$
$$BP = (HR \times SV) \times TPR$$

The physiologic control of blood pressure is complex and involves all those factors that regulate cardiac performance and vascular resistance. Blood pressure control involves two processes in general: 1) a fast-acting process via vascular reflexes and 2) a slow-acting process via fluid volume adjustment. Under resting conditions, the pressure is regulated mostly by the arteriolar resistance. With exercise, however, alterations in stroke volume and heart rate (cardiac output, cardiac performance) may play a more significant role.

Peripherally placed baroreceptors (mechanoreceptors) and chemoreceptors exist to maintain a steady blood pressure. Baroreceptors are stretch receptors located in the carotid sinus and in the proximal aortic arch. These receptors have neural connections with the cardiovascular center of the medulla via cranial nerves IX and X, respectively. The frequency of baroreceptor discharge decreases when the blood pressure decreases and vice versa. For example, during a hypotensive episode the baroreceptor discharge rate decreases, the cardiovascular center of the medulla becomes less inhibited, there is an increase in vasoconstrictor activity mediated by the medulla, and, subsequently, there is an increase in total peripheral resistance and blood pressure. If the stimulus is intense, there will be increased inotropic and chronotropic influences on the heart in addition to vasoconstriction. These responses will increase cardiac output and blood pressure.

Baro- and chemoreceptors act as sensors to regulate steady blood pressure.

The chemoreceptors are the carotid and aortic bodies. They respond to decreases in PO_2 and arterial pH. Stimulation of these receptors will increase ventilation but only minimally increase peripheral resistance. Their role in the overall control of the cardiovascular system is small.

The chemoreceptors respond to arterial PO_2 and pH.

Flow Resistance

Changes in total peripheral vascular resistance (TPR) via activation of the sympathetic nervous system are an important governing factor over blood flow and blood pressure. The TPR can be calculated as follows:

Defining TPR

$$TPR = \frac{AP - CVP}{Q_T} \times 80$$

where

TPR = total peripheral resistance (dynes $\times$ sec $\times$ cm^{-5})

AP = mean systemic arterial pressure (mm Hg)
= diastolic pressure + ⅓ pulse pressure

CVP = central venous pressure (mm Hg)

Q_T = cardiac output (liters/min)

80 = a conversion factor

TPR is normally 1000–1600 dynes $\times$ sec $\times$ cm^{-5}.

The Hagan-Poiseuille relationship defines flow resistance.

The normal TPR is 1000–1600 dynes $\times$ sec $\times$ cm^{-5}.

In addition to changes in the diameter of resistance vessels, the resistance to blood flow is also related to vessel length and blood viscosity by the Hagan-Poiseuille relationship:

$$Resistance = \frac{8 \times vessel\ length \times viscosity}{\pi \times vessel\ radius^4}$$

Since resistance is related to the fourth power of the vessel radius, it is clear that small changes in vessel diameter can have a large effect on TPR. Blood viscosity is also important and is related to: 1) the hematocrit, 2) blood flow, and 3) vessel diameter.

The hematocrit is the most important factor governing viscosity. The viscosity of whole blood is about 3.5 times that of water. A decrease in hematocrit to half normal causes the viscosity of blood to decrease to 2 times that of water. Anemia, therefore, improves the rheologic properties of blood. Polycythemic states have an adverse effect on blood flow. When the hematocrit is raised to 70% above normal, the viscosity of blood increases to 20 times normal.

Anemia improves the flow properties of blood.

Cellular Energetics

ATP is the metabolic fuel for most cellular processes.

ATP is the metabolic fuel for most active cellular processes, including active transport, muscle contraction, and protein synthesis. Hydrolysis of the ter-

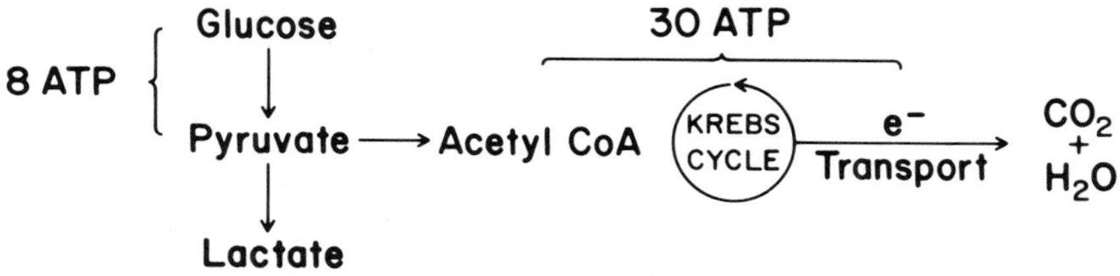

Aerobic Glycolysis $\longrightarrow$ 10 ATP - 2 ATP used =   8 ATP net

Aerobic Krebs Cycle, e⁻ Transport $\longrightarrow$ = 30 ATP net

$\qquad\qquad\qquad\qquad\qquad$ TOTAL = 38 ATP net

38 x 8,000 cal/mole = 304,000 cal

$\qquad\qquad\qquad\qquad$ = 1/2 combustion energy

$\qquad\qquad\qquad\qquad$ = 50% eff.

Anaerobic Glycolysis $\longrightarrow$ 4 ATP - 2 ATP used =   2 ATP net

2/38 = 5% of energy produced

$\qquad$ = < 3% eff.

FIGURE 1.6   Energy yield by glucose combustion under aerobic and anaerobic conditions.

minal phosphate ester group of ATP yields about 8000 cal/mole. This energy becomes available to do cellular work.

In the Embden-Meyerhof glycolytic pathway, 10 moles of ATP is produced per mole of glucose metabolized under aerobic conditions (Figure 1.6). Two moles of ATP is consumed in the reactions catalyzed by hexokinase and phosphofructokinase. The net ATP produced, therefore, under aerobic glycolysis is 8 moles of ATP per mole of glucose. With the additional metabolism of pyruvate to acetyl-CoA and, ultimately, carbon dioxide and water, via the Krebs cycle and the electron transport chain of the mitochondria, an additional 30 moles of ATP is produced per mole of glucose.

Under aerobic conditions 38 moles of ATP is produced by the combustion of 1 mole of glucose. This aerobic process is 50% efficient.

Under aerobic conditions, therefore, the total ATP produced by the metabolism of 1 mole of glucose is 38 moles. This is equivalent to 38 moles times 8000 cal/mole, or 304,000 cal produced by the metabolism of 1 mole of glucose. This represents about 50% of the total combustion energy in glucose. Thus the overall aerobic process is about 50% efficient.

▬ Oxygen Consumption and Delivery

In general, alterations in oxygen (O_2) delivery to cells and utilization by cells may cause abnormalities in cellular metabolism that can cause death. Four factors are involved in normal tissue O_2 consumption:

There are four factors controlling tissue O_2 consumption.

1) respiratory function, 2) erythrocyte O_2 transport, 3) capillary perfusion, and 4) cellular utilization of the O_2 delivered. Any or all of these factors may be deranged in shock.

Respiratory Function

The ability of the lungs to oxygenate blood is obviously a vital process. Shock may cause progressive pulmonary insufficiency, especially if sepsis coexists. Respiratory failure following shock and trauma is called the adult respiratory distress syndrome (ARDS). There are numerous other names for this condition, including shock lung, post-traumatic pulmonary insufficiency, pump lung, and traumatic lung, to name a few.

Pulmonary failure may occur following shock.

Pulmonary insufficiency following shock has three components: 1) progressive hypoxemia, 2) decreased lung compliance, and 3) decreased functional residual capacity (FRC).

Pulmonary failure following shock has three components.

Progressive hypoxemia may be caused by: 1) hypoventilation, 2) altered diffusion capacity, 3) ventilation-perfusion abnormalities, or 4) increased pulmonary shunting. Most patients in shock have adequate alveolar ventilation and thus normal or low PCO_2, unless the shock is severe and prolonged. Likewise, diffusion capacity plays but a minor role in the hypoxemia that may accompany shock.

The causes of hypoxemia

Normally, there is a balance between alveolar ventilation and the blood supply to those alveoli. When alveolar ventilation decreases there is a compensatory or matching decrease in the perfusion of these alveoli. In shock there may be mismatching of ventilation and perfusion. Two abnormalities may exist: 1) adequate ventilation with decreased perfusion ("dead space ventilation") or 2) adequate perfusion with decreased ventilation ("increased intrapulmonary shunting"). Dead space ventilation usually does not cause hypoxemia but can influence the ability to eliminate carbon dioxide.

Increased shunting usually causes hypoxemia. Pathologic shunting occurs when the alveoli are filled with blood, debris, or edema fluid or are involved by pneumonia or atelectasis. Blood then perfuses nonventilated areas. Normally a physiologic shunt of 3–5% of the cardiac output exists because of the bronchial and Thebesian veins. In shock complicated by ARDS the ventilation-perfusion mismatch may increase the shunt fraction greatly. When this fraction is greater than 25%, mechanical ventilatory support is usually needed.

Lung compliance may decrease during shock. Compliance is the change in lung volume per change in inflation pressure. An estimate of pulmonary and chest wall compliance may be made by dividing the tidal volume by the peak respiratory pressure. Both of these parameters can be measured at the bedside. Normal compliance is about 100–200 ml/cm H_2O.

A decrease in FRC also contributes to the pulmonary insufficiency of shock. The FRC is the volume of gas in the lungs at end-expiration. It measures about 2 liters in the adult. A decrease in FRC will result in alveolar collapse, progressive atelectasis, and increased shunting.

Ventilation-perfusion abnormalities and shunting are the major causes of hypoxemia after shock.

Normal compliance is 100–200 ml/cm H_2O.

A decrease in FRC will cause more shunting.

Erythrocyte O_2 Transport

The affinity of hemoglobin for O_2 is defined by the oxyhemoglobin dissociation curve, which is sigmoidal in shape (Figure 1.7). It relates the O_2 tension of blood to the saturation of hemoglobin by O_2. The steep part of the curve occurs at those levels of PO_2 found at the capillary bed. A shift in the curve will

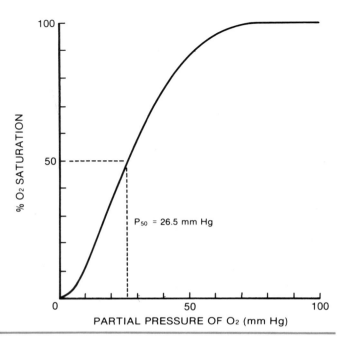

FIGURE 1.7 The oxyhemoglobin dissociation curve is sigmoidal in shape and relates the O_2 tension of blood to the saturation of hemoglobin by O_2. The normal P_{50} is 26.5 mm Hg.

A rightward shift in the oxyhemoglobin dissociation curve increases O_2 delivery to the tissues.

Normal P_{50} is 26.5 mm Hg.

Factors causing a rightward shift in the curve

The Bohr effect

have its greatest effect at the capillary level. A rightward shift in the curve means a decrease in O_2 affinity, and more O_2 is released by hemoglobin to the tissues. This may be expressed as an increase in P_{50}, or the O_2 tension necessary to saturate 50% of the hemoglobin with O_2. The P_{50} is normally 26.5 mm Hg at a body temperature of 37.5°C and a blood pH of 7.4.

Several factors can cause a rightward shift in the curve and increase P_{50}. These include a decreased pH, increased temperature, increased PCO_2, increased erythrocyte 2,3-diphosphoglycerate (2,3-DPG), and increased erythrocyte ATP and aldosterone. Thyroxine, cortisol, increased pH, and young cell age can also increase P_{50} indirectly by increasing levels of 2,3-DPG.

The major control of the O_2 affinity for hemoglobin is by changes in blood pH (the Bohr effect). A change in the concentration of 2,3-DPG in response to pH is a slower compensatory process. Changes in blood pH during shock have an acute influence on the position of the oxyhemoglobin dissociation curve. Acidemia improves the unloading of O_2 to peripheral tissues.

Capillary Perfusion

Oxygen delivery to tissues depends mostly on the degree of capillary perfusion. Adequate tissue oxygenation can be calculated by measuring O_2 consumption or can be estimated using the mixed venous PO_2, or $P\bar{v}O_2$. The $P\bar{v}O_2$ is the partial pressure of O_2 in mixed venous blood, that is, blood sampled from the pulmonary artery using a Swan-Ganz catheter. It normally measures 35–40 mm Hg. In a critically ill patient a decrease in the $P\bar{v}O_2$ means that more O_2 is being removed by the tissues. If the $P\bar{v}O_2$ decreases below 30 mm Hg, then tissue oxygenation is inadequate. In other words, the tissues are extracting more O_2 to meet their metabolic demands during a period of circulatory insufficiency.

Mixed venous PO_2 $(P\bar{v}O_2)$

Oxygen consumption (VO_2) is directly related to cardiac output as follows:

$$VO_2 = (CaO_2 - C\bar{v}O_2) \times Q_T \times 10$$

where

How to calculate O_2 consumption (VO_2)

VO_2 = O_2 consumption (ml/min)
CaO_2 = O_2 content of arterial blood (vol%)
$C\bar{v}O_2$ = O_2 content of mixed venous blood (vol%)
Q_T = cardiac output (liters/min)

CaO_2 and $C\bar{v}O_2$ are defined as follows:

$$CaO_2 = (PaO_2 \times 0.003) + (Hb \times 1.39)SaO_2$$
$$C\bar{v}O_2 = (P\bar{v}O_2 \times 0.003) + (Hb \times 1.39)S\bar{v}O_2$$

where

PaO₂ = partial pressure of O_2 in arterial blood (mm Hg)
P$\bar{v}$O₂ = partial pressure of O_2 in mixed venous blood (mm Hg)
Hb = hemoglobin concentration (g/100 ml)
SaO₂ = oxyhemoglobin saturation in arterial blood (%)
S$\bar{v}$O₂ = oxyhemoglobin saturation in mixed venous blood (%)
0.003 = solubility coefficient of O_2 dissolved in solution
1.39 = amount of O_2 bound to hemoglobin (ml/g)

Oxygen consumption can be calculated by measuring: 1) cardiac output, 2) arterial and mixed venous blood gas analysis, and 3) hemoglobin concentration.

In general, changes in the FIO_2 have little effect on the ultimate O_2 consumption, whereas changes in cardiac output and hemoglobin concentration have major effects. The VO_2 normally measures about 195–280 ml/min for a 70-kg man.

Case Study

A 60-year-old man is admitted to the intensive care unit with an acute upper gastrointestinal hemorrhage. With the patient breathing room air the following database is obtained: Hb = 8 g/100 ml; PaO_2 = 95 mm Hg; $P\bar{v}O_2$ = 40 mm Hg; SaO_2 = 97%; $S\bar{v}O_2$ = 75%; Q_T = 4 liters/min. Using the above formulas:

$$CaO_2 = 11.1 \text{ vol\%}$$
$$C\bar{v}O_2 = 8.6 \text{ vol\%}$$
$$VO_2 = 100 \text{ ml/min}$$

The patient is placed on 50% O_2 so that PaO_2 = 250 mm Hg and SaO_2 = 99%. The other data are unchanged. Now the calculated values are:

Clinical calculation of VO_2

$$CaO_2 = 11.8 \text{ vol\%}$$
$$C\bar{v}O_2 = 8.6 \text{ vol\%}$$
$$VO_2 = 128 \text{ ml/min}$$

The patient is then transfused 5 units of blood so that Hb = 15 g/100 ml and Q_T = 5.6 liters/min. The other data remain the same. Now:

$$CaO_2 = 21.4 \text{ vol\%}$$
$$C\bar{v}O_2 = 15.8 \text{ vol\%}$$
$$VO_2 = 314 \text{ ml/min}$$

Increases in inspired O_2 have only a small effect on O_2 consumption by tissues. The clinical message is that in order to maintain good tissue O_2 consumption the cardiac output and the hemoglobin concentration must be maintained.

With the above background it is now possible to calculate the amount of pulmonary shunt in any critically ill hypoxemic patient. The following data are required in order to calculate the shunt: 1) PAO_2,

2) PaO_2, 3) CaO_2, and 4) $C\overline{v}O_2$. The shunt equation is:

The pulmonary shunt equation

$$\frac{Q_S}{Q_T} = \frac{CcO_2 - CaO_2}{CcO_2 - C\overline{v}O_2}$$

where

Q_S = shunt blood flow (liters/min)
CcO_2 = O_2 content of pulmonary capillary blood (vol%)
= $(0.003 \times PAO_2) + (Hb \times 1.39)SAO_2$
PAO_2 = alveolar O_2 pressure (mm Hg)
SAO_2 = oxyhemoglobin saturation of pulmonary capillary blood (%)

For $PaO_2 > 150$ mm Hg, the modified shunt equation can be used, since both the arterial and the pulmonary capillary hemoglobin are fully saturated. This equation is easier to calculate manually:

$$\frac{Q_S}{Q_T} = \frac{(PAO_2 - PaO_2)0.003}{(CaO_2 - C\overline{v}O_2) + (PAO_2 - PaO_2)0.003}$$

Case Study

A 30-year-old woman undergoes a common bile duct exploration for suppurative cholangitis. She is septic and intubated in the intensive care unit. The following database is obtained while she has been breathing 100% O_2 for 15 minutes: PaO_2 = 125 mm Hg; SaO_2 = 99%; Hb = 15 g/100 ml; $P\overline{v}O_2$ = 40 mm Hg; $S\overline{v}O_2$ = 75%; $PaCO_2$ = 36 mm Hg; SAO_2 = 100%. The calculated values are:

Clinical use of the shunt equation

PAO_2 = $PB - PH_2O - PaCO_2$
= $760 - 47 - 36$
= 677 mm Hg
CcO_2 = 22.9 vol%
CaO_2 = 21.0 vol%
$C\overline{v}O_2$ = 15.8 vol%

Therefore:

$$\frac{Q_S}{Q_T} = \frac{22.9 - 21.0}{22.9 - 15.8}$$
$$= 0.27$$

The pulmonary shunt is 27%. Approximately 10 cm of positive end-expiratory pressure (PEEP) is added to the ventilatory support. Repeat labs are unchanged except the PaO_2 = 225 mm Hg and the SaO_2 = 100%. Then:

PAO_2 = 677 mm Hg
CaO_2 = 21.5 vol%
$C\overline{v}O_2$ = 15.8 vol%

Therefore:

$$\frac{Q_S}{Q_T} = \frac{(677 - 255)0.003}{(21.5 - 15.8) + (677 - 225)0.003}$$
$$= 0.19$$

The pulmonary shunt is now decreased to 19% with PEEP therapy.

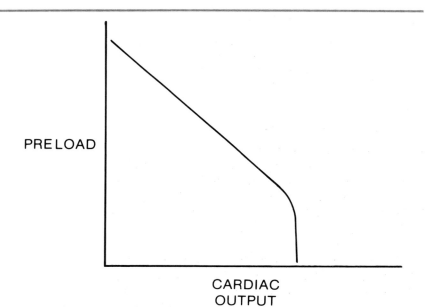

CARDIAC
OUTPUT

FIGURE 1.8   The systemic function curve is a graphic way to portray venous return function. It relates the functional dependence of preload on cardiac output. In general, an increase in cardiac output causes a decrease in preload. Reprinted with permission from Kreis DJ Jr. Shock (Part I): Pathophysiology. Curr Rev Respir Dis 6:61, 1983.

Cellular Utilization

An increase in metabolic rate and energy requirements causes an increase in O_2 utilization by cells. Shock causes an intracellular energy crisis by uncoupling the mitochondria from normal ATP production. Whether this metabolic block in shock is due to decreased O_2 delivery or decreased O_2 utilization by cells or both is unknown at present.

▭ Integration of the Cardiac and Vascular Systems

We have reviewed in this chapter those factors that control heart rate, stroke volume, blood pressure, and vascular resistance. Under normal conditions the cardiovascular system is a closed loop with the right and left sides of the circulation connected in series. Over any period of time, therefore, the cardiac output must equal the venous return.

Cardiac output equals venous return.

The venous return is caused by a pressure gradient between the peripheral circulation and the right atrium. This gradient is called the mean systemic pressure and measures 7 mm Hg in the dog. The value in humans is unknown. It represents the pressure that would be present in the circulation if blood flow stopped and blood were transferred from the arterial side to the venous side until pressure was uniform.

Mean systemic pressure is 7 mm Hg in the dog.

The ventricular function curve is a graphic way to portray cardiac function. It relates the functional dependence of cardiac performance (cardiac output) on filling pressure or preload (CVP, mean PCWP). The reverse relationship exists as well. The systemic function curve is a graphic way to portray venous return function. It relates the functional dependence of preload on cardiac performance (Figure 1.8). In general, an increase in cardiac output causes a decrease in preload, and a decrease in cardiac output causes an increase in preload. The point where the graph intersects the y-axis (cardiac output equals zero) is the mean systemic pressure.

The systemic function curve relates the preload as a function of cardiac output.

Blood volume and vascular resistance regulate the systemic function curve.

The main factors that influence the position of the systemic function curve are: 1) blood volume and 2) vascular resistance. The ratio of arterial-to-venous capacitance also plays some role but not acutely.

The axes of the systemic function curve may be reversed arbitrarily so that they are similar to the ventricular function curve (Figure 1.9). A decrease in blood volume will shift the systemic function curve to the left, whereas an increase in blood volume will shift the curve to the right. Changes in vascular re-

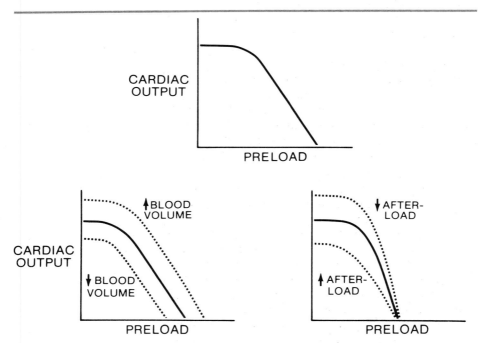

FIGURE 1.9   The axes of the systemic function curve may be reversed so that they are similar to the ventricular function curve. The main factors that influence the position of the systemic function curve include: 1) the blood volume and 2) the vascular resistance. An increase in blood volume will shift the curve upward and to the right. A decrease in blood volume will have the opposite effect. A decrease in vascular resistance (afterload) will rotate the curve clockwise, whereas an increase in resistance will have the opposite effect. Reprinted with permission from Kreis DJ Jr. Shock (Part I): Pathophysiology. Curr Rev Respir Dis 6:62, 1983.

sistance alter the curve in a more complex manner. In general, a decrease in resistance will rotate the curve clockwise, whereas an increase in resistance will rotate the curve counterclockwise relative to the x-axis intercept. This is so because changes in vascular resistance, unlike blood volume, do not alter the mean systemic pressure.

The cardiac and systemic function curves can be plotted on the same graph (Figure 1.10). The point of intersection between both curves represents the equilibrium point in overall cardiovascular function at any given time. Homeostatic mechanisms tend to maintain a steady state about this point.

The cardiac and systemic function curves serve a practical conceptual purpose. They can be applied as a pictorial representation of cardiovascular physiology. Formulating such a schema will clarify the altered physiology, normal homeostatic mechanisms, and effects of therapeutic intervention in the treatment of shock. This will be done in the subsequent chapters.

The cardiac and systemic function curves can be integrated on the same graph.

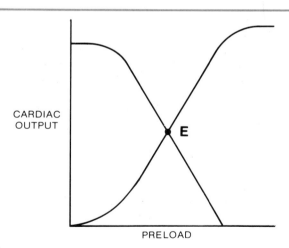

CARDIAC OUTPUT

E

PRELOAD

FIGURE 1.10   The ventricular and systemic function curves can be integrated on the same graph. The point of intersection (E) between both curves represents the equilibrium point in overall cardiovascular function at any given time. Homeostatic mechanisms tend to maintain a steady state about this point. Reprinted with permission from Kreis DJ Jr. Shock (Part I): Pathophysiology. Curr Rev Respir Dis 6:61, 1983.

Annotated Bibliography

Beal JM (ed). Critical Care for Surgical Patients. Macmillan, New York, 1982.

A recent textbook on critical care medicine.

Berk JL, Sampliner JE (eds). Handbook of Critical Care. Little, Brown, Boston, 1982.

An excellent, physiologic approach to intensive care medicine with a clinical orientation as well.

Berne RM, Levy MN. Cardiovascular Physiology. C. V. Mosby, St. Louis, 1972.

Contains a detailed review of the systemic and ventricular function curves.

Braunwald E. Regulation of the circulation. N Engl J Med 290:1124–1129, 1420–1425, 1974.

A succinct review of cardiovascular physiology.

Braunwald E, Ross J Jr, Sonnenblick EH. Mechanisms of Contraction of the Normal and Failing Heart. Little, Brown, Boston, 1976.

An extensive account of cardiac structure and function in health and disease.

Cowley RA, Trump BF (eds). Pathophysiology of Shock, Anoxia, and Ischemia. Williams & Wilkins, Baltimore, 1982.

A monumental book on the pathophysiology of shock. The book stresses detailed physiology and basic science.

Gorlin R. Practical cardiac hemodynamics. N. Engl J Med 296:203–205, 1977.

A brief, clear discussion of hemodynamic parameters.

Kelman GR. Applied Cardiovascular Physiology. Butterworths, Boston, 1977.

An excellent review of cardiovascular physiology.

Little RC. Physiology of the Heart and Circulation. Year Book, Chicago, 1977.

An excellent review of cardiovascular physiology.

Rushmer RF. Structure and Function of the Cardiovascular System. W. B. Saunders, Philadelphia, 1972.

This book contains a concise discussion of those factors that control blood pressure.

Additional Bibliography

Braunwald E. Determinants and assessment of cardiac function. N Engl J Med 296:86–89, 1977.

Guyton AC, Young DB (eds). Cardiovascular Physiology III (International Review of Physiology, Vol. 18). University Park Press, Baltimore, 1979.

Kaley G, Altura BM. Microcirculation, Vol. I. University Park Press, Baltimore, 1977.

Najarian JS, Delaney JP (eds). Critical Surgical Care. Stratton Intercontinential, New York, 1977.

Parker JO, Case RB. Normal left ventricular function. Circulation 60:4–12, 1979.

Shepro D, Fulton GP. Microcirculation as Related to Shock. Academic Press, New York, 1968.

Sonnenblick EH, Strobeck JE. Derived indexes of ventricular and myocardial function. N Engl J Med 296:978–982, 1977.

Wells R (ed). The Microcirculation in Clinical Medicine. Academic Press, New York, 1973.

Shock: An Overview 2

Overview

This chapter reviews the etiology, diagnosis, patho-biology, and treatment of shock. Shock is not a disease but rather a clinical syndrome caused by circulatory insufficiency and inadequate tissue per-fusion. There are three main causes (cardiogenic, hematogenic, and vasogenic) related to changes in three main physiologic parameters. (cardiac output, blood volume, and vascular resistance). There is much interplay and overlap between the clinical etiology and the underlying physiologic abnormal-ity. In general, the treatment of shock involves: 1) establishing normovolemia and 2) improving cardiac performance.

▨ Definition

Shock may best be defined as a clinical syndrome caused by circulatory insufficiency and inadequate tissue perfusion.

▨ Etiology

The first use of the term shock is credited to James Lotta in 1795. Clowes in 1568, Weismann in 1719, and de Garengeot in 1723 all recognized the clinical syndrome of shock and thought it was due to a for-eign body in the wound or the blood. Until the early part of this century, shock was considered by most physiologists and physicians to result from a pri-mary dysfunction in the nervous system. Travers in 1826 stated that "shock is a species of functional concussion by which the influence of the brain over the organ of circulation is deranged or suspended."

Historical background

Goltz in 1863 gave the first experimental evidence that shock may be due to vasomotor failure. The theory of exhaustion of the vasomotor center as a cause of shock was popularized in Crile in 1897. Henderson in 1908 thought shock was caused by hyperventilation, which causes hypocarbia (the acapnea theory). Cannon and Bayliss in 1919 thought that shock was due to some sort of humoral depressant agent.

Blalock in 1934 was the first to classify shock in physiologic terms. He described four causes of shock: 1) cardiogenic, due to pump failure; 2) hematogenic, in which there is a decrease in blood volume; 3) vasogenic, in which vasodilatation occurs due to humoral agents; and 4) neurogenic, in which vasodilatation is due to altered vascular tone. Since both vasogenic and neurogenic causes of shock in Blalock's classification are due to primarily to alteration in peripheral vascular resistance, neurogenic causes should be considered a subset of vasogenic causes. In summary, therefore, there are three main physiologic causes of shock: 1) cardiogenic, 2) hematogenic, and 3) vasogenic, or altered peripheral vascular resistance (Table 2.1).

In common practice physicians recognize five clinical forms of shock. Each of these forms develops because of one of the above causes. The clinical forms of shock are: 1) cardiogenic shock, 2) hypovolemic or hemorrhagic shock (hematogenic), 3) septic shock (vasogenic), 4) neurogenic shock (vasogenic), and 5) anaphylactic shock (vasogenic). Septic shock, neurogenic shock, and anaphylactic shock are all subsets of vasogenic shock.

Blalock's classification of shock

The three causes of shock

The five clinical forms of shock

TABLE 2.1   The Causes of Shock

Blalock's (1934) Classification	*Current Classification*
Cardiogenic: pump failure	Cardiogenic
Hematogenic: decrease in blood volume	Hematogenic
Vasogenic: vasodilatation due to humoral agents	Vasogenic: altered peripheral vascular resistance
Neurogenic: vasodilatation due to altered vascular tone	Septic Neurogenic Anaphylactic

There is much interplay between the clinical form of shock and its underlying physiologic causes. More than one cause of shock may be operating at the same time.

Clinical Form	Physiologic Mechanism
Cardiogenic	Altered Cardiac Output
Hemorrhagic	Altered Blood Volume
Septic	Altered Vascular Resistance
Neurogenic	

These is much interplay between the clinical form of shock and the underlying physiologic causes. For example, in cardiogenic shock the main cause may be pump failure. There may also be an element of hypovolemia (hematogenic cause) contributing to the shock syndrome. Similarly, prolonged hemorrhagic shock may cause myocardial failure. In the clinical situation it is important to remember that more than one cause of shock may be operating at the same time.

Interplay between physiologic cause and clinical form of shock

Cardiogenic Shock

Primary causes of pump failure include: 1) acute myocardial infarction (AMI), 2) cardiac dysrhythmias, 3) congestive heart failure, 4) carditis and cardiomyopathies, and 5) congenital heart disease. Cardiogenic shock may complicate an AMI in about 15% of patients.

Etiologies of cardiogenic shock

Secondary causes of pump failure include those factors that cause a mechanical obstruction to blood flow or cardiac function. These include: 1) pulmonary embolism, 2) cardiac tamponade, 3) vena cava syndrome, 4) tension pneumothorax, 5) intracardiac tumor or thrombus, and 6) dissecting aortic aneurysm.

Hematogenic Shock

Etiologies of hemato-
genic shock

The causes of hematogenic shock include losses of: 1) whole blood volume, as in hemorrhage; 2) plasma volume, as in burns and peritonitis; and 3) extravascular, extracellular fluid volume, as in bowel obstruction and colitis.

Vasogenic Shock

Etiologies of vasogenic
shock

The clinical forms of vasogenic shock include: 1) septic shock, 2) neurogenic shock, and 3) anaphylactic shock. The ultimate agent responsible for altered vascular resistance in sepsis is not known. Neurogenic shock can be caused by: 1) spinal cord trauma, 2) neurogenic reflex, or 3) anesthetic agents.

Anaphylactic shock is the most severe form of an allergic reaction and may cause death. The large amount of histamine released during an anaphylactic reaction causes profound vasodilatation, hypotension, and shock. Since this syndrome is primarily an immunologic phenomenon, the reader is referred to standard internal medicine and immunology textbooks for a detailed review of this subject.

▓ Diagnosis

Shock is usually easily recognized. The classical findings are hypotension, a weak and rapid pulse, shallow and rapid respiration, altered mental status, skin pallor and coldness, diminished urine production, and acidemia. There are deviations from this picture, however, particularly in sepsis.

Hypotension is the
cardinal sign of circu-
latory failure.

Patients in shock usually have a systolic blood pressure less than 90 mm Hg. In a previously normotensive patient a decrease in systolic pressure to less than 80–90 mm Hg indicates circulatory insufficiency. In a previously hypertensive patient, however, a decrease in blood pressure of 50 mm Hg would indicate hypotension. This is true especially in the geriatric age group, in whom systolic hypertension is common. In sepsis, on the other hand, hypertension may be noted initially.

The heart rate in shock is variable. Most patients have tachycardia (heart rate above 110) as a compensatory mechanism to improve cardiac output. Bradycardia (heart rate below 60) occasionally is noted, as in an AMI. Except in moribund patients most patients in shock have tachypnea due to sympathoadrenal stimulation. Body temperature is variable. One of the early findings in sepsis, particularly in the newborn and geriatric populations, is hypothermia rather than fever. The cutaneous manifestations of shock may vary from cold, clammy skin (as in hemorrhagic and cardiogenic shock) to warm, dry skin (as in early septic shock). Cyanosis may occur.

Most patients in shock are tachycardic.

Alterations in cerebral functioning in shock can range from anxiety to coma. Cortical neurons are irreversibly damaged after 5 minutes of hypoxia. Elderly patients are more sensitive to cerebral hypoxia. In addition, cerebrovascular disease limits the ability to autoregulate cerebral blood flow. The elderly patient is most susceptible to the cerebral effects of hypotension.

Altered mental status in shock

▩ Pathophysiology and Homeostasis

Regardless of etiology the hallmark of shock is inadequate tissue blood flow. At present there is no exact way to clinically monitor microcirculatory flow during shock. The parameter used most commonly to indicate shock is the blood pressure. Hypotension can result from changes in either cardiac output or peripheral vascular resistance or both. The factors controlling blood pressure can be summarized graphically (Figure 2.1).

Several factors control blood pressure.

Several homeostatic mechanisms exist normally to counteract circulatory insufficiency. These mechanisms are more efficient in the young adult than in the child or the elderly individual. There are three main homeostatic adjustments in shock: 1) cardiovascular, 2) hormonal, and 3) blood volume. All three tend to improve cardiac output and elevate blood pressure. They do so concurrently as an integrated homeostatic response. These three components will next be discussed.

Homeostatic mechanisms in shock

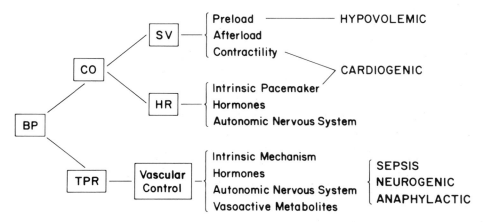

FIGURE 2.1   The various clinical forms of shock cause hypotension mainly by alteration in the mechanisms shown. BP, blood pressure; CO, cardiac output; TPR, total peripheral vascular resistance; SV, stroke volume; HR, heart rate. Adapted with permission from Rushmer RF. Structure and Function of the Cardiovascular System. W. B. Saunders, Philadelphia, 1972, p 169.

Cardiovascular Adjustments

In shock there occur compensatory mechanisms throughout the cardiovascular system. For example, in trauma the initiation of these mechanisms results from afferent neuron input from the injured area to the vasomotor center of the medulla.

The role of barore-
ceptors as sensors of
circulatory failure

The baroreceptors act as the sensors of circulatory insufficiency in acute hypotension. The baroreceptors decrease their inhibition of the cardiovascular center of the medulla during hypotension. This causes an augmented sympathetic output from this center. This results in: 1) vasoconstriction of the arteriolar resistance vessels, 2) vasoconstriction of the venous capacitance vessels, and 3) increased heart rate and cardiac contractility. If hypoxemia or acidemia is also present, the sympathetic discharge may be augmented further by impulses from the carotid and aortic body chemoreceptors.

Redistribution of
blood flow in shock

In shock there is a preferential redistribution of blood flow to the brain and the heart. Vasoconstriction is most pronounced in skin, kidney, skeletal muscle, and splanchnic vascular beds but negligible in the coronary and cerebral circulations. The coronary arteries may actually dilate.

Vasoconstriction of the venous capacitance vessels causes an "autotransfusion" of about 10% of the total blood volume, or about 500 ml in the 70-kg adult. This augments cardiac preload and thus stroke volume, cardiac output, and blood pressure.

Vasoconstriction causes an "autotransfusion" of about 500 ml in the adult.

Hormonal Adjustments

Shock activates the neuroendocrine axis. Endocrine stimulation causes: 1) vascular pressor changes and 2) fluid volume changes. Endogenous vasopressors include epinephrine, norepinephrine, dopamine, angiotensin, and vasopressin (ADH). Glucocorticoids may also play a role in regulating vascular tone. Aldosterone and ADH secretion are important in preserving blood volume.

Endocrine stimulation results in vasopressor effects and conservation of water and salt.

Volume Adjustments

Vasoconstriction during shock causes a decrease in capillary perfusion and capillary filtration pressure. Fluid moves from the interstitium to the intravascular space according to Starling's law of capillary exchange. Total blood volume is expanded and cardiac preload is enhanced.

F. D. Moore and associates have extensively studied the phenomenon of plasma refill. In adult volunteers, after a bleed of 500–1000 ml of blood the initial rates of plasma refill are 90–120 ml/h for 2 hours. Plasma refill averages 40–60 ml/min for the first 6–10 hours. Refill is complete in 30–40 hours. Of particular importance is the finding that the volume of new plasma added to the intravascular compartment equals the volume of shed whole blood. The degree of plasma refill can vary greatly with the severity of hemorrhage. For example, in severe hemorrhagic shock from trauma the rate of plasma refill may approach 1000 ml in the first hour.

Plasma refill supports blood volume and preload.

Pathology in Shock: Organ Level

Cardiac lesions are common even in the absence of coronary artery disease.

About 45% of patients dying from noncardiogenic shock will have pathologic cardiac lesions despite the lack of coronary artery disease. These lesions are indistinguishable from cardiac ischemic lesions and include focal necroses and hemorrhages, particularly in the subendocardial areas. Cardiac cell nuclei may disappear and fatty degeneration may occur.

Renal lesions in shock

The renal lesions in shock include: 1) acute tubular necrosis (ATN, common), 2) fibrin thrombi in glomeruli (less common), and 3) bilateral cortical necrosis (rare). If shock is treated promptly, ATN is usually a reversible lesion. The proximal and distal convoluted tubules are the most sensitive to ischemia. Hyalin casts, pigment casts, and focal necrosis may be found.

Lung lesions in shock

Pulmonary lesions in shock may include edema fluid, hemorrhage, hyalin membranes, fat emboli, and microthrombi. In hemorrhagic shock per se, however, pulmonary lesions are not routinely observed.

Brain lesions in shock

Brain cells may be swollen or necrotic. The typical brain lesion in shock includes fibrin thrombi in venules with surrounding hemorrhage. These lesions occur commonly in the cerebral gray matter and basal ganglia.

The liver in shock can show dilatation of the hepatic sinusoids due to cellular aggregates, hepatic cell plate disruption, and areas of necrosis.

The adrenal glands in shock may have areas of necrosis, hemorrhage, or fibrin thrombi.

Gastrointestinal lesions are rare in shock in humans but common in canine experimental models. These lesions include diffuse mucosal and submucosal hemorrhages as well as areas of focal ulceration. These findings are typical of ischemic enterocolitis.

Pathology in Shock: Cellular Level

Summary: the cell in shock

Morphologic intracellular changes occur in shock. These include cellular edema and disruption of mitochondria. The exact relationship between abnormal cellular structure and abnormal cellular function remains to be defined.

Shock alters membrane transport function. Hemorrhagic shock causes a decrease in the resting membrane potential of muscle. This results in an influx of sodium and water into the cell and an efflux of potassium out of the cell. Adenosine triphosphate levels decrease in liver, kidney, and muscle. Sodium and potassium transport across the cell membrane is under the control of an adenosine triphosphatase (ATPase) pump. The activity of this ATPase pump increases in shock to compensate for the increasing levels of intracellular sodium. More ATP is used up. ATP and cyclic adenosine monophosphate (cyclic AMP) levels decrease. Cellular membranes become less responsive to various hormones, including catecholamines, insulin, and glucagon, and lysosomal enzymes are released into the cell. These may hydrolyze membranes, ribonucleic acids, and phosphate esters. Calcium may also serve as an intracellular toxin in this process. There is ultimately disruption of cell architecture and function. Lysosomal enzymes can also leak into the circulation and damage other organs.

Cellular Energetics

During the anoxic stress of circulatory insufficiency and shock, the Krebs cycle and electron transport chain process are inhibited. ATP production may become solely dependent on the anaerobic glycolytic process. During aerobic glycolysis 6 of the 10 moles of ATP produced per mole of glucose metabolized are formed via the respiratory chain oxidation of two dihydronicotinamide adenine dinucleotides (NADH coenzyme). Under anaerobic conditions the NADH generated cannot be utilized by the mitochondria to produce ATP. Two moles of ATP is consumed during the glycolytic process. The net production of ATP via anaerobic glycolysis is only 2 moles of ATP per mole of glucose. This represents about 5% of the energy produced during aerobic glucose combustion and represents an efficiency of less than 3%.

Anaerobic glycolysis yields only 2 moles of ATP per mole of glucose metabolized. This causes a cellular energy crisis in shock.

Carbohydrate Metabolism

Caloric values:
Carbohydrate =
4 cal/g
Protein = 4 cal/g
Fat = 9 cal/g

The American diet is high in carbohydrate, much of which is converted to fat. This has certain advantages since the caloric value of fat (9 cal/g) is twice that of either carbohydrate (4 cal/g) or protein (4 cal/g). Glucose can also be stored as glycogen in the liver and muscle. In a 70-kg man about 150 g of glycogen is stored in muscle and about 75 g is stored in liver. About 20 g of glucose is present in the extracellular fluid. The energy extractable from muscle and liver glycogen and from extracellular glucose totals about 1000 cal.

The energy available from glucose stores is about 1000 cal.

In shock the normal metabolism of glucose to water and carbon dioxide is inhibited. The result is an increased production of lactic acid (the end product of anaerobic glycolysis) and a decreased production of ATP. The body's initial response is to mobilize glucose via the breakdown of hepatic and muscle glycogen. This process, called glycogenolysis, requires ATP.

Epinephrine stimulates glycogenolysis and inhibits the release of insulin.

Epinephrine released during shock stimulates liver and muscle adenyl cyclase. This enzyme breaks down ATP to cyclic AMP. Cyclic AMP stimulates in turn various protein kinases, which cause the enzymatic degradation of glycogen into glucose-1-phosphate. Glucose then becomes available as a fuel. Epinephrine also inhibits insulin release by the pancreas. Glucagon too is released in shock; it also stimulates adenyl cyclase activity and thus augments glycogenolysis, but only in liver. The effects of epinephrine and glucagon cause an early rapid hyperglycemia in shock. This is in the 250 mg% range. This compensatory metabolic response, however, is short-lived, since the glycogen stores are totally depleted after 2 hours of shock.

Glycogen stores are depleted after 2 hours of shock.

Gluconeogenic pathways are activated in shock.

The production of new sugar, called gluconeogenesis, is a further compensatory mechanism needed to produce glucose and ultimately ATP. Gluconeogenesis occurs mainly in the liver and to a lesser degree in the kidney. The amount of glucose produced by gluconeogenesis may be 10 times that produced by glycogenolysis. The metabolic substrates available for the production of new sugar include: 1) amino acids, 2) glycerol, and 3) lactic acid. In humans there is no metabolic pathway that can utilize the two carbons of the acetyl group of acetyl-CoA in the formation of new net sugar. The acetyl-CoA produced by fatty acid catabolism, however, may enter the Krebs cycle and contribute to ATP production.

Protein Metabolism

Shock causes the catabolism of protein and a state of negative nitrogen balance. The liver is able to use most amino acids in the generation of new sugar. This process is under the control of glucocorticoids, which cause: 1) protein breakdown into amino acids, 2) increased hepatic uptake of amino acids, and 3) increased activity of the enzymes responsible for hepatic gluconeogenesis. They further influence the metabolism of fat and sugar by: 4) increasing lipolysis and 5) decreasing glucose utilization in extrahepatic tissues. The protein catabolic effects of glucocorticoids occur mostly in skeletal muscle protein rather than visceral protein.

Glucocorticoids stimulate protein catabolism in skeletal muscle.

The amino acids released into the blood from skeletal muscle are converted by liver enzymes to either acetyl-CoA or intermediates of the Krebs cycle. There are 20 different pathways of amino acid oxidation and entry into the Krebs cycle for the 20 different amino acids. Most amino acids are glycogenic and their carbon skeletons can be converted into new glucose.

Released amino acids are metabolized in the liver.

Alanine is the main amino acid released by skeletal muscle during protein catabolism and contributes most to hepatic gluconeogenesis. Alanine catabolism plays a major role in the formation of new glucose by the liver in shock. In addition, alanine is involved in a mechanism whereby the glucose utilized by muscle is in part salvaged by the liver. This is known as the glucose-alanine-glucose cycle. Muscle catabolizes glucose to pyruvate, which is then converted to alanine. Alanine enters the blood and is reconverted into pyruvate and, ultimately, into glucose via hepatic gluconeogenesis.

Alanine contributes most to hepatic gluconeogenesis.

The alanine cycle is a pathway for glucose salvage.

Leucine is the one amino acid that is solely ketogenic. It cannot be utilized in the formation of

Leucine is the only amino acid that cannot form new net sugar.

new net sugar. This is so because its carbon skeleton is converted to acetyl-CoA. Five other amino acids are both glycogenic and ketogenic: isoleucine, lysine, phenylalanine, tyrosine, and tryptophan.

Lipid Metabolism

Lipolysis is under hormonal control.

The catabolism of lipid, or lipolysis, releases free fatty acids and glycerol into the circulation. Both epinephrine and glucagon stimulate the adenyl cyclase system of adipose tissue, which in turn, via cyclic AMP, activates triglyceride lipase. Glucocorticoids also have a stimulating effect on lipolysis.

Glycerol is a substrate for hepatic gluconeogenesis.

Glycerol is a substrate for gluconeogenesis. It is transported to the liver and converted to triose phosphate and ultimately glucose. Free fatty acids, on the other hand, are not gluconeogenic except for the 3-carbon fragment of a fatty acid having an odd number of carbon atoms. These acids are catabolized by the liver and other organs (heart, kidney, muscle) to acetyl-CoA.

Lactate Metabolism

Lactic acid is produced in great quantity during shock, particularly from ischemic skeletal muscle. The increased production of lactic acid contributes significantly to the metabolic acidemia of shock. Arterial pH may drop below 7.1. Hyperventilation cannot compensate for this serious degree of acid load.

When blood lactate levels exceed 12 mM in shock, the mortality rate is greater than 90%.

Various investigators have correlated serum lactate levels with prognosis of recovery from shock. When levels are greater than 12 mM, the mortality rate is greater than 90%. Blood lactate levels, therefore, may serve as a guide to the severity of cellular metabolic derangement during shock.

The Cori cycle is a pathway for glucose salvage.

The liver is capable of metabolizing lactate and can utilize it to produce new sugar. This is called the Cori cycle. Ischemic skeletal muscle metabolizes glucose to lactate. Lactate enters the circulation and is converted to pyruvate in the liver. Pyruvate can then be converted to new glucose. Like the glucose-alanine-glucose cycle, the Cori cycle acts as a salvage pathway for the regeneration of glucose utilized in muscle glycolysis.

Acid-Base Status

About 75% of patients in hemorrhagic shock will have a metabolic acidosis. Often a mixed acid-base disorder is observed. Apart from the effects of acidemia on respiratory drive, shock itself induces a central, neurally regulated hyperventilation. This causes a respiratory alkalosis. The arterial pH may be normal or in the alkalotic range when initial blood gases are obtained. If shock is severe this compensatory mechanism will fail. Acidemia will result mostly because of accumulation of lactic acid. There are two other causes of this acidemia in shock: one involves proteolysis and the other lipolysis.

In shock there may be an initial respiratory alkalosis.

Lactate acidemia is the main cause of acidemia in shock.

ATP depletion in shock will inhibit gluconeogenesis. The amino acids released into the circulation by protein catabolism will not be metabolized adequately by the liver. The resulting aminoacidemia may contribute to the acidemia of shock.

Aminoacidemia in shock

The by-products of free fatty acid catabolism include the ketone bodies, acetoacetate, and β-hydroxybutyrate. During normal metabolism ketone bodies are produced in low levels when the major metabolic fuel is sugar. In shock the liver and other tissues cannot oxidize these ketone bodies. Ketosis and acidemia may result.

Ketosis in shock

▬ Patient Monitoring

It is important to discuss which parameters should be monitored during shock. Some, like blood pressure, are obviously vital, whereas others, like blood lactate levels, are not. Monitoring techniques are a way to access homeostatic mechanisms, pathophysiologic reactions, and response to therapy.

Monitoring is a vital way to assess physiologic reactions and response to therapy.

A list of those specific areas that should be monitored in any critically ill patient in shock is presented in Table 2.2.

TABLE 2.2   Parameters to be Monitored in Shock

	Parameter	*Monitoring Devices*
Circulatory function	Blood pressure	Arterial catheter
	Pulse	EKG
	Preload	CVP catheter
	Preload	Swan-Ganz catheter
	Cardiac output	Swan-Ganz catheter
Respiratory function	ABG	Arterial catheter
Renal function	Urine output	Foley catheter
	BUN	Blood sample
	Creatinine	Blood sample
	Urine sodium	Urine sample
Volume	CVP	CVP catheter
	PCWP	Swan-Ganz catheter
	Urine output	Foley catheter
	Blood pressure	Arterial catheter
	Pulse	EKG
	Hematocrit	Blood sample
	BUN	Blood sample
Acid-base status	Arterial blood gas with pH	Arterial catheter
Electrolyte status	Serum electrolytes	Blood sample
Coagulation profile	PT	Blood sample
	PTT	Blood sample
	Platelet count	Blood sample
Temperature status	Temperature	Rectal thermistor

Reprinted with permission from Kreis DJ Jr. Shock (Part II): Therapy. Curr Rev Respir Dis 6:66–71, 1984.

Circulatory Function

Blood pressure should be monitored using an arterial catheter.

It may be difficult to hear Korotkoff sounds during shock using a sphygmomanometer. A more accurate method of blood pressure monitoring is by direct arterial cannulation. The radial artery is used most commonly. It may be cannulated using a number 20- or 18-gauge plastic catheter placed either percutaneously or by arterial cutdown. Repeated percutaneous attempts at cannulation should be avoided so that the artery is not injured.

Method of radial artery cutdown

In radial artery cutdown, a transverse incision is made on the volar wrist medial to the styloid process of the radius. This usually corresponds to the proximal volar wrist skin crease. The artery is usually easily identified and can, therefore, be cannulated under direct vision. The intracath can then be connected to a pressure transducer and a display panel for continuous blood pressure display. Other

Other arteries that may be cannulated

arterial sites may be used but are less desirable. These

include the ulnar, brachial, superficial temporal, dorsalis pedis, posterior tibial, and, rarely, the femoral arteries. The complications of arterial cannulation include thrombosis, distal ischemia, and antegrade air embolism.

Heart rate is important since it is directly related to cardiac output. Sinus tachycardia is the rule in most forms of shock, although other arrhythmias can occur. This is most true during shock associated with myocardial infarction. Heart rate and rhythm can be continuously monitored using the electrocardiogram (EKG).

> A continuous EKG should be displayed and monitored.

Monitoring the EKG is essential. Severe cardiac dysrhythmias may be acutely discovered and treated. A complete 12-lead EKG should also be taken at periodic intervals to assess the development of cardiac ischemia or infarction.

All patients in shock require a central venous pressure (CVP) catheter. The normal CVP is less than 10 cm H_2O. The CVP is identical to the right atrial pressure, and since the tricuspid value is low in resistance it approximates the right ventricular end-diastolic pressure.

> A CVP line should be placed.

The CVP does not reflect accurately the left heart filling pressure and function. More important than the absolute, isolated CVP reading is the response of the CVP to volume loading. In this manner the CVP can be used as a guide to fluid therapy.

> The CVP can guide fluid therapy.

If the patient is in shock and the CVP is low (for example, less than 5 cm H_2O), then fluids may be administered in an attempt to augment preload. If after several fluid challenges the CVP rises to 15 cm H_2O and the patient still remains hypotensive, then some component of myocardial dysfunction is usually also contributing to the shock syndrome. At this point the administration of digoxin and other inotropic agents, such as dopamine, would be warranted. Fluids should not usually be pushed if the CVP is above 15 cm H_2O, since this may precipitate heart failure and pulmonary edema. In patients with preexisting cardiopulmonary disease, a Swan-Ganz catheter is usually necessary to accurately monitor preload of the left ventricle so as to avert iatrogenic congestive heart failure and pulmonary edema.

The CVP catheter can be placed via several venous routes. These include the antecubital (basilic,

> Method of CVP catheter placement

cephalic), subclavian, internal jugular, and even external jugular veins. It is important that the catheter be situated in the superior vena cava (confirmed by chest x-ray) and that there be good respiratory dynamics. The CVP catheter can be attached to either a manometer for intermittent measurements or a transducer with display panel for continuous CVP readings. The antecubital and jugular routes are preferred. The subclavian route, although popular, should be reserved for the most emergent circumstances, since it carries a substantial risk of pneumothorax. This is especially true if the insertion is being attempted by a novice.

The subclavian route should be used only emergently because of risk of pneumothorax.

The internal jugular vein is usually easily cannulated. There are several methods of internal jugular vein cannulation. At the Yale-New Haven Hospital the following method is commonly used: The patient is positioned with legs elevated. The head is turned to the side opposite that being cannulated. The carotid artery is retracted medially. Using a 14-gauge Jelco catheter attached to a 10-ml syringe with suction being applied on the syringe, the catheter is inserted on the medial border of the sternocleidomastoid muscle about one-half the way up from the suprasternal notch. The catheter is directed posterior to the muscle and advanced slowly with the tip aiming just medial to the ipsilateral nipple. Once the vein is punctured, the catheter is advanced into it, the syringe and metal needle are removed, and a 16-gauge, 8-inch long intracath is threaded through the Jelco catheter into the superior vena cava. Other approaches to the internal jugular vein include an approach lateral to the sternocleidomastoid muscle and another approach that bisects the sternal and clavicular heads of the sternocleidomastoid muscle.

How to cannulate the internal jugular vein

In like fashion, the subclavian vein can be cannulated. This is accomplished at the midpoint of the clavicle, making sure that the needle hugs the inferior clavicular border and that the direction of the needle is initially at the cricoid and not at the suprasternal notch. If the first attempt fails, the needle can be guided more inferiorly at the midpoint between the cricoid and the suprasternal notch. If this fails also, which is rare, the needle may be directed at the suprasternal notch, but this probably carries a greater risk of pneumothorax.

How to cannulate the subclavian vein

The Swan-Ganz balloon flotation catheter

measures left-sided cardiac filling pressures and function. Any patient in shock with a component of myocardial dysfunction, significant chronic obstructive pulmonary disease, or renal failure should be monitored with a Swan-Ganz catheter because of the inaccuracy of CVP measurements in these patients. The triple-lumen Swan-Ganz catheter is preferred so that serial cardiac output measurements can be made by the thermodilution technique.

Indication for Swan-Ganz catheter placement

The Swan-Ganz catheter can easily be positioned in the pulmonary artery at the bedside without fluoroscopy by monitoring the pressure at the distal port. Various veins may be catheterized. These include the basilic, cephalic, brachial, internal and external jugular, subclavian, and femoral veins. The balloon is inflated once the catheter is near the right atrium. The catheter has marked calibrations of 10 cm. The tip is near the right atrium at 15 cm when the internal jugular or subclavian vein is used, at 40 cm when the right basilic vein is used, at 50 cm when the left basilic vein is used, and at 30 cm when the femoral vein is used. With the balloon inflated and while observing the continuous pressure trace, the catheter is sequentially advanced through the right atrium, the right ventricle, and into the pulmonary artery (usually the right). The catheter is further advanced into the "wedge" position. This occurs when the balloon diameter exceeds that of a smaller pulmonary artery branch. If the balloon is subsequently deflated at this point, the pulmonary artery trace and pressure will be observed. Reinflation causes the catheter to float distally, once again into the wedge position. The catheter position should next be confirmed by chest x-ray.

Placement of the Swan-Ganz catheter at the bedside

In the wedge position, the pressure recorded at the distal port represents the pulmonary vein and capillary pressure. This pulmonary capillary wedge pressure (PCWP) measures 6–12 mm Hg normally. The PCWP is important for it represents: 1) pressure in the pulmonary veins, which is a major factor in the development of pulmonary edema, and 2) pressure in the left atrium (LAP). The PCWP approximates the LAP and, in the absence of either significant mitral valvular disease or left ventricular dysfunction, the left ventricular end-diastolic pressure (LVEDP). With left ventricular failure, that is, when LVEDP is greater than 15 mm Hg, the PCWP

The PCWP measures 6–12 mm Hg normally.

The PCWP reflects changes in LAP and LVEDP.

and the LAP may be less than the actual LVEDP and thus may not actually measure the LVEDP directly. The PCWP will, nonetheless, reflect changes in the LVEDP.

The PCWP measures the LAP and can be used clinically to monitor left ventricular preload. It is an accurate guide to fluid therapy and volume loading of the left heart in patients in shock.

The PCWP is used to monitor left ventricular preload and fluid therapy.

Regardless of etiology, shock may be associated with hypovolemia. The PCWP may be low. Volume loading to increase the PCWP to 15–18 mm Hg will, in most patients, maximize ventricular preload and cardiac performance. At levels of PCWP above 15–18 mm Hg further volume loading will usually not increase stroke volume or cardiac output, since at these levels of preload the ventricular function curve is already flat.

A PCWP above 18 mm Hg may cause pulmonary edema.

At PCWP levels greater than 18 mm Hg the incidence of pulmonary congestion increases. Frank pulmonary edema will result in most patients at a PCWP of 30 mm Hg. At this level the pulmonary capillary pressure exceeds the plasma colloid osmotic pressure (normally about 25 mm Hg). Fluid will shift from the capillaries into the pulmonary interstitial space and eventually into the alveoli (classical pulmonary edema). A corollary to the above is that most patients in shock with an elevated PCWP (greater than 15–18 mm Hg) usually do not need additional volume. These patients, therefore, would require some combination of the following types of drugs in order to support blood pressure and to improve ventricular performance: inotropic agents, vasopressors, preload reduction (diuretics), and afterload reduction (vasodilators).

The complications of Swan-Ganz catheterization

The complications of Swan-Ganz catheterization include: 1) pulmonary infarction, 2) pulmonary artery rupture, 3) balloon rupture, 4) cardiac dysrhythmias, 5) thromboembolism, 6) infection, and 7) catheter knotting. Since there is potential for pulmonary artery rupture and pulmonary infarction, the PCWP should be measured infrequently. Usually the pulmonary artery end-diastolic pressure (PADP) is only slightly higher than the mean PCWP, by 1–3 mm Hg. In most cases, therefore, the PADP can be used to approximate the PCWP. The balloon may thus be kept deflated, and the catheter will be positioned more proximally in the pulmonary artery.

Inflating the balloon may rupture the pulmonary artery.

The PADP can be used to approximate the PCWP in most cases.

The PADP may be measured and displayed continuously on a monitor.

Several conditions preclude the PADP from accurately approximating the LAP and the LVEDP. These are: 1) increased pulmonary vascular resistance and pulmonary hypertension, 2) mitral stenosis, 3) right bundle branch block with delayed right ventricular ejection, 4) advanced aortic regurgitation, 5) decreased pulmonary vascular compliance, and 6) chronic left ventricular dysfunction. In these conditions, therefore, it would be important to measure the PCWP intermittently.

Conditions in which the PADP may not accurately reflect LAP and LVEDP

The triple-lumen Swan-Ganz catheter may be used for cardiac output determinations at the bedside. The thermodilution technique is most commonly used today. It is a modification of the dye-dilution technique. Ten milliliters of 5% dextrose in water at either ambient or ice-cold temperature is injected through the proximal port. The catheter has a built-in thermistor, which senses the decrease in temperature that occurs distally in the pulmonary artery. Using a commercially available computer, the cardiac output is electronically calculated and displayed. The use of cold dextrose solution (0–4°C) has a better reliability than ambient temperature solution. Three determinations are made at one time and an average value is calculated. The reproducibility of the measurement is usually within 5%.

How to measure the cardiac output using the Swan-Ganz catheter

By the above method the cardiac output of the right ventricle can be calculated. This is a helpful hemodynamic parameter to measure, particularly in the patient in cardiogenic shock or postoperatively after heart surgery. Since cardiac output does not represent ventricular filling, simultaneous determination of CVP, PADP, or PCWP should be made to determine the need for volume therapy. A ventricular function curve can be developed thereby at the bedside by recording cardiac output at different levels of ventricular preload.

A ventricular function curve can be constructed at the bedside using the Swan-Ganz catheter.

Respiratory Function

The rate of breathing offers a quick way to assess respiratory function and the need for immediate ventilatory support. If the patient in shock has agonal

Evaluate breathing pattern.

or labored respirations or is tachypneic (rate above 35 per minute), then endotracheal intubation should be accomplished without delay. Sometimes this is necessary even before the results of blood gas analysis are available. It will ensure an adequate airway for ventilatory exchange and arterial oxygenation.

Obtain an ABG.

Arterial blood gases (ABG) should be obtained promptly on any patient in shock. Significant hypoxemia or hypercarbia mandates oxygen therapy and mechanical ventilation.

Obtain a chest x-ray.

A chest x-ray should be obtained to further assess cardiopulmonary status. This is usually done after the patient has been intubated and central lines have been placed so that the position of these tubes and lines can be checked at the same time.

Renal Function

Normal urine output is 0.5–1.0 ml/kg/h.

A Foley catheter must be placed so that hourly urine outputs can be accurately measured. An adequate urine output for an adult is about 30 ml/h or 0.5–1.0 ml/kg/h. Hourly urine outputs are an easy way to assess renal perfusion and function.

The blood urea nitrogen (BUN) and creatinine levels should be obtained, both as a baseline and to evaluate for the existence of underlying renal disease.

Evaluating renal function

Any patient with either oliguria (urine output < 20 ml/hr) or polyuria (urine output > 100 ml/hr) needs to be worked up with renal function studies. These involve evaluating: 1) glomerular filtration, 2) tubular function, and 3) concentrating ability.

A 1-hour creatinine clearance test can be used to approximate glomerular filtration rate (GFR). GFR is calculated as follows:

How to calculate GFR

$$ GFR = \frac{U_{cr} \times V}{P_{cr}} $$

where

GFR = glomerular filtration rate (ml/min)
U_{cr} = concentration of creatinine in urine (mg/ml)
V = flow rate of urine (ml/min)
P_{cr} = concentration of creatinine in plasma (mg/ml)

Thus, to calculate GFR one can collect urine for 1

hour and measure urine flow rate and urine creatinine and draw a blood sample for plasma creatinine. Normal GFR is about 100 ml/min. In shock this may decrease to 40 ml/min. Values of GFR below 30 ml/min indicate renal failure.

Tubular function can be measured by the degree of sodium reabsorption. Urine sodium concentration normally measures about 15–40 mEq/liter. An elevated urine sodium concentration would indicate an impairment in sodium conservation and renal insufficiency. Tubular function can also be evaluated by measuring the urine-to-plasma sodium ratio or the urine-to-plasma creatinine ratio. The normal urine-to-plasma sodium level is about 0.1. With tubular injury more sodium is excreted and this ratio will elevate. The normal urine-to-plasma creatinine level is about 100. With tubular damage less creatinine is excreted and this ratio will fall to below 10.

How to assess tubular function

Renal concentrating ability can be estimated by measuring the ratio of urine-to-plasma osmolality. Normally this ratio is greater than 1.3. In renal failure dilute urine may be produced, and this ratio will decrease to less than 1.1.

How to evaluate concentrating ability

Volume Status

It is experimentally possible to measure red blood cell mass, plasma volume, and extracellular fluid volume. To measure these parameters clinically during the initial management of the patient in shock is impractical and unnecessary. In order to evaluate volume status an overall clinical assessment must be made, including history, physical examination, vital signs, urine volume, hematocrit, BUN, CVP, and PCWP measurements. As previously discussed, the CVP or the PCWP can be used to guide volume therapy. Although they are not direct measures of volume, the changes seen in these parameters are a good indicator of the patient's volume status.

Volume status assessment involves an integration of many factors.

Acid-Base Status

Arterial pH should be promptly measured so that sodium bicarbonate therapy can be started as needed. Unless the patient is moribund when first seen, bi-

Measure arterial pH.

carbonate therapy should await the results of the pH measurement, since patients in shock are sometimes initially alkalotic.

Electrolyte Status

Measure serum electrolytes.

Serum electrolytes should be determined promptly. If the patient is acidemic, then hyperkalemia may be found. If the patient has been on diuretics at home, then hypokalemia may be found. Hyponatremia and hypocalcemia may also be observed.

Calculate the anion gap.

When time permits, the anion gap should be calculated. It is estimated by subtracting the sum of the chloride and bicarbonate levels from the sodium level. The anion gap normally measures below 12–14 mEq/liter. Small elevations to the 15- to 16-mEq/liter range are sometimes found with respiratory alkalosis. Elevation above this level usually indicates metabolic acidemia.

An elevated anion gap would be expected in severe shock with lactic acidemia. Other clinical causes of an anion gap acidosis include uremia, diabetes, and certain drug overdoses, such as alcohol, phenformin, and paraldehyde.

Coagulation Status

Measure PT, PTT, and platelet count.

Patients in shock may have an altered coagulation profile. It is important to measure the prothrombin time (PT), the partial thromboplastin time (PTT), and the platelet count. This is particularly important in patients with underlying hepatic dysfunction or sepsis. An altered coagulation profile may herald the onset of the disseminated intravascular coagulation (DIC) syndrome, and further tests should then be performed to help document the presence of DIC. These tests include the fibrinogen level, fibrin split products, and thrombin time.

Temperature Status

Insert a rectal temperature probe.

Body temperature is a vital sign that should not be forgotten when managing the patient in shock. A rectal temperature probe will suffice. Aberration in body

temperature may indicate the beginning of septicemia. Hyperthermia increases the general metabolic
rate and should be corrected. Hypothermia depresses cardiac function and may cause dysrhythmias and cardiac arrest and therefore should be recognized and treated.

▬ Treatment

Certain guidelines exist in the resuscitation of the
patient in shock (Table 2.3). They may be applied
universally to the critically ill patient in shock, to
the trauma victim, and during cardiopulmonary resuscitation (CPR). The priorities form a schema for
orderly resuscitation efforts. They are commonly
called the ABCs of resuscitation: Airway, Breathing,
and Circulation. Adherence to these priorities in the
order stated is important for patient survival.

ABCs of treatment

General Measures

A brief, pertinent history should be obtained either
from the patient, the patient's family, witnesses, or
the nursing staff. Often this is impossible initially,

Obtain a quick history,
if possible, while ex-
amining the patient.

TABLE 2.3   ABCs of Resuscitation

Airway	Maintaining airway patency may involve: 1) Suctioning or removing debris, blood, or vomitus from oropharynx 2) Lifting jaw and tongue forward (chin lift) 3) Nasotracheal or endotracheal intubation 4) Cricothyroidotomy
Breathing	Maintaining ventilation may involve: 1) Use of Ambu bag 2) Use of mechanical respirator
Circulation	Maintaining circulation may involve: 1) Digital pressure on all external bleeding sites 2) Volume loading with crystalloid and/or blood 3) Military anti-shock trousers (MAST suit) 4) Inotropic agents such as dopamine 5) Vasopressors (rarely)

and the physician is forced to make diagnostic and therapeutic decisions based on physical examination only. Particular initial attention should be directed at the vital signs, the patient's breathing ability and pattern, mental status, gross neurologic function, skin color, skin temperature, and examination of the heart, lungs, abdomen, and extremities. This initial assessment usually takes less than 1 minute (Table 2.4).

Establish an airway if there is respiratory distress.

If there is respiratory distress, an airway should be established immediately and 100% oxygen should be started. If the patient is in hemorrhagic shock, several large-bore, 14-gauge Jelco catheters should be placed. In trauma victims the upper extremities are preferred rather than the lower extremities because of the possibility of injury to the great veins beneath the diaphragm. The patient's legs should be elevated. This causes an autotransfusion of about 500 ml and will thereby augment preload. A true Trendelenberg's position should be avoided, since this may increase carotid sinus flow and pressure and cause an unwarranted peripheral vasodilation. A CVP catheter should next be placed and measured. A Foley catheter should be inserted into the bladder, unless the patient has obvious urethral injury. Blood samples are drawn for type and crossmatch, blood count, glucose, BUN, electrolytes, PT, PTT, and platelets. An ABG should be obtained. An EKG monitor is attached to the patient and a full cardiogram obtained.

Insert large IVs.

Insert a CVP line. Insert Foley catheter. Obtain blood samples.

Run an EKG. Obtain a chest x-ray.

TABLE 2.4   Checklist for the Orderly Management of Any Critically Ill Patient in Shock

1) Secure airway
2) Insert at least two large-bore IVs
3) Start crystalloid solution
4) Send baseline blood work
5) Insert Foley catheter
6) Insert CVP line
7) Obtain chest x-ray
8) Obtain EKG
9) Consider the MAST suit
10) Insert nasogastric tube, if indicated
11) Start antibiotics, if indicated
12) Start steroids, if indicated

Reprinted with permission from Kreis DJ Jr. Shock (Part II): Therapy. Curr Rev Respir Ther 6:66–71, 1984.

A portable chest x-ray will further assess the heart and lungs and confirm the position of the CVP catheter.

Respiratory Function

Of prime importance is the initial evaluation of respiratory function, because of the rapid deleterious effects of cerebral hypoxia. When in doubt, it is always better to place an airway and later remove it rather than procrastinate while deciding whether or not the patient needs artificial ventilatory support. Indeed, the tragic situation sometimes occurs in which the patient's cardiovascular system survives shock but the patient's brain does not. Securing the airway is always step number one. This is usually accomplished by endotracheal intubation using a number 7 or 8 endotracheal tube in the adult. If intubation is difficult or impossible, then an emergent cricothyroidotomy is performed. A formal tracheostomy should be avoided since, even when performed in an emergent situation by an experienced surgeon, the time involved is prohibitive, usually about 5 minutes. A cricothyroidotomy can usually be performed in less than 1 minute and is preferred.

First priority: secure the airway.

Either intubate or perform a cricothyroidotomy. Avoid formal tracheostomy.

Once an airway is established, the presence of bilateral breath sounds should be sought, since the endotracheal tube may have been advanced too far down one mainstem bronchus. During the initial resuscitation the patient should be placed on 100% oxygen administered by hand bagging using an Ambu bag. Once stabilized, the patient should be placed on a volume respirator. The PaO_2 should be maintained at about 65–70 mm Hg. It is usually unnecessary to raise the PaO_2 much above this level, since there is little to be gained in hemoglobin saturation and oxygen delivery to tissues by such a maneuver. The initial inspired oxygen concentration should be set at 100%. This may be decreased in time depending on subsequent ABG determination. Ideally the FIO_2 should be lowered to 40–50% as soon as possible so as to prevent the development of pulmonary oxygen toxicity. This complication is related to both the dose of oxygen and the duration of administration.

Administer 100% O_2 initially.

Maintain the PaO_2 at about 70 mm Hg.

Use of volume-cycled respirator

Intermittent mandatory ventilation

The respiratory rate should be set at 10 or 12 breaths per minute. The tidal volume should be 10–15 ml/kg body weight or about 1000 ml for the average adult. Either continuous mechanical ventilation or intermittent mandatory ventilation (IMV) may be used. IMV allows the alert patient to breathe spontaneously in addition to receiving the set number of respirations. The main disadvantage of IMV is that the patient may expend more energy and work harder breathing through an artificial airway because of its attendant increased resistance to air flow.

The use of sedative drugs and pancuronium in the intubated patient

Intubated patients often require sedation to control spontaneous respiratory rates. With ongoing shock, sedation is dangerous because of the side effect of hypotension. Once the emergent situation has passed and the patient becomes hemodynamically stable, sedative drugs like morphine sulfate (1–4 mg IV every hour as needed) or diazepam (2–4 mg IV every hour as needed) may be used to control activity. The occasional patient may need to be paralyzed in order to effect adequate ventilation and respiratory control. This is accomplished by using a loading dose of pancuronium (0.05–0.1 mg/kg IV). An average adult would require about 6–8 mg pancuronium IV as a loading dose followed by doses of 1–2 mg IV every hour as needed.

The use of PEEP

If the intubated patient remains hypoxemic despite an FIO_2 of greater than 50–60%, positive end-expiratory pressure (PEEP) should be added in increments starting at 5 cm H_2O. PEEP causes an increase in PaO_2, functional residual capacity, and static lung compliance. It expands atelectatic alveoli and may decrease physiologic shunting. Its major advantage is that the FIO_2 may be subsequently decreased to more safe levels while maintaining an adequate PaO_2 on PEEP.

PEEP may cause a pneumothorax and a decreased cardiac output.

Two major drawbacks of PEEP are the complications of pneumothorax and decreased cardiac output. With PEEP less than 15 cm H_2O, the incidence of pneumothorax is about 7%. This incidence doubles as PEEP approaches 25 cm H_2O. One of the earliest warning signs of possible pneumothorax is an elevation in the pressure generated by the volume respirator. PEEP may decrease cardiac output particularly in the hypovolemic patient. It does so by elevating the intrapleural pressure. This compresses the central great veins and causes a decrease in cardiac preload. PEEP levels of 10 cm H_2O or less are usually well tolerated.

PEEP levels below 10 cm H_2O are usually well tolerated.

Circulatory Function

Once the respiratory function has been evaluated and treated, attention can be directed at treating the circulatory insufficiency of shock. There are two main avenues of treatment: 1) reestablishment of normovolemia and 2) improvement in cardiac performance (Table 2.5). These two functions are interrelated. Often improving the volume status will result in improvement in cardiac functioning due to the influence of preload on stroke volume.

Reestablish normovolemia. Improve cardiac performance.

The objective of volume loading (or deloading in hypervolemic states) is to optimize ventricular preload. This involves administering fluid volume until the plateau phase of the ventricular function curve is reached. This occurs for most adults at a CVP of 12–15 cm H_2O or at a PCWP at 15–18 mm Hg. If shock remains refractory to adequate fluid volume, then attention should be directed at improving: 1) cardiac inotropy and 2) vascular tone.

The objective of volume loading is to optimize cardiac preload. This occurs at a CVP of 12–15 cm H_2O or at a PCWP of 15–18 mm Hg.

Volume Status Hypovolemia must be corrected so that there exists an adequate effective blood volume and cardiac preload. The CVP and PCWP can be used to guide fluid therapy. If these parameters are not available, then the blood pressure, pulse rate, and urine output measurements may suffice initially.

TABLE 2.5 Two Main Avenues of Treatment of Shock

1) Reestablish normovolemia
   a) Volume loading (commonly)
   b) Volume unloading (occasionally)

2) Improve cardiovascular performance
   a) Inotropic agents
   b) Sodium bicarbonate
   c) Calcium chloride
   d) MAST suit
   e) Vasopressor agents (rarely)

Reprinted with permission from Kreis DJ Jr. Shock (Part II): Therapy. Curr Rev Respir Dis 6:66–71, 1984.

Use lactated Ringer's
in the initial treatment
of shock.

Much has been debated and written about the choice of fluid needed in the resuscitation of shock. At present there is much convincing experimental and clinical data to support the use of a balanced salt solution, like lactated Ringer's, in the initial treatment of shock. Ringer's solution approximates plasma electrolyte composition and osmolality. As such, it is an excellent fluid choice and is effective in increasing CVP, improving hemodynamics, maintaining oxygen consumption, and correcting the acidemia of severe shock. In a Wiggers model of hemorrhagic shock in the dog, Shires and associates have demonstrated improved survival in those animals given lactated Ringer's solution and shed blood. Indeed, the survival rate beyond 24 hours was 70% for those dogs receiving lactated Ringer's plus shed blood, but only 20% for those receiving shed blood alone.

In hemorrhagic shock
use lactated Ringer's
and blood.

The use of lactated Ringer's in hemorrhagic shock has two major advantages: 1) it decreases the need for blood transfusion and 2) it improves the rheologic properties of blood by decreasing blood viscosity via hemodilution. Some investigators have criticized the use of lactated Ringer's on two accounts: 1) that the metabolic lactic acidemia of shock may be aggravated by lactated Ringer's infusion and 2) crystalloid use may precipitate adult respiratory distress syndrome (ARDS). It has been shown, however, that by improving the hemodynamic profile and flow properties of blood during shock, lactated Ringer's solution improves and corrects the acidemia of severe shock. As the circulation improves, blood lactic acid levels fall. Furthermore, several clinical studies have failed to demonstrate any correlation between the use of lactated Ringer's in resuscitation and the development of ARDS.

Criticisms leveled
against the use of
lactated Ringer's are
unfounded.

How much lactated
Ringer's to administer
initially

In the initial treatment of shock, 1–2 liters of lactated Ringer's solution should be administered in 15 minutes unless there is obvious pulmonary edema. Usually this will stabilize the hemodynamic profile if the patient is hypovolemic. In the trauma victim or in the hemorrhaging patient, this fluid challenge serves two functions. First, it will allow time for accurate blood typing and crossmatching. Second, if the hemodynamic profile becomes unstable after this volume load, then ongoing hemorrhage must be suspected. This is particularly true if the preload, either CVP or PCWP, remains low.

Caution must be used when using CVP readings as a guide to fluid therapy. A patient may have a low CVP reading and yet be in left ventricular failure. Conversely, a patient may have an elevated CVP reading and normal left ventricular function. It is obviously more important to observe the response of the CVP to increments of volume loading rather than to concentrate on isolated readings. If a 250-ml fluid bolus markedly elevates the CVP without improving the hemodynamic profile (blood pressure, pulse rate, urine output), the patient may be in borderline fluid overload. Likewise, if fluid bolus therapy improves the hemodynamic profile and raises the CVP, but only transiently, then more fluid volume can be administered.

How to give fluid bolus therapy

In the anemic patient in shock or with ongoing hemorrhage, volume therapy should include blood transfusions. Blood should be properly typed and crossmatched. Only rarely should type-specific blood or uncrossmatched type O negative blood be used. In the trauma victim with hemorrhage, fresh whole blood should ideally be used. This is rarely available and, therefore, component therapy with packed red blood cells and fresh frozen plasma (FFP) should be used. About 1 unit of FFP should be given for each 4–5 units of red blood cells. This will avert the potential for coagulopathy from dilution of clotting factors during massive transfusions.

The use of blood products to support volume

The hematocrit may be used as an indicator of the type of blood component to give. If the hematocrit is greater than 35, then FFP or whole blood should be given. If the hematocrit is between 30 and 35, then whole blood should be given. If the hematocrit is less than 30, then packed red blood cells should be given along with appropriate amounts of FFP. Ideally, in the bleeding patient the hematocrit should be maintained at 30–35, since at this level the rheologic properties of blood flow are enhanced at the same time that the oxygen-carrying capacity of blood remains adequate.

The hematocrit may be used as a guide to the type of blood component to give.

Maintain the hematocrit at 30–35.

Colloid use should be restricted in the initial resuscitation of the patient in shock. It should be remembered that FFP, like blood, causes a definite risk of hepatitis transmission. Salt-poor albumin, in either 12.5- or 25-g aliquots or as a 5% solution in saline, may be given to selected patients. Albumin is expensive but does not carry a significant hepatitis

Colloid use should be restricted.

The indications for albumin therapy are limited.

risk. Its use should be limited to: 1) the nonhemorrhaging patient with hematocrit greater than 35, 2) those patients who require strict salt restriction, as in the cirrhotic, and 3) the hypoproteinemic patient. The theoretical advantage of albumin infusion, namely, the maintenance of normal plasma colloid osmotic pressure, is unfounded. For example, one study has shown that, despite the administration of 250 g of albumin during therapy, the total protein and albumin blood levels were not significantly higher than for those not given albumin. Albumin may leak into the pulmonary parenchyma if there exists a significant capillary leak. This may aggravate pulmonary congestion and insufficiency.

Albumin infusion may aggravate pulmonary congestion.

If albumin is unavailable, then human plasma protein fraction (plasmanate, plasmatein) may be used as colloid therapy in selected patients. This contains 5% human plasma proteins and has a minimal hepatitis risk.

Dextran can no longer be recommended as a volume agent.

Dextran, although once a popular plasma expander, can no longer be recommended because of the risks of anaphylaxis, increased bleeding tendency, and difficulty with blood crossmatching that are associated with its use.

Cardiac Status   If shock remains refractory to adequate volume loading, then therapy should be directed at the heart and peripheral vessels.

There are various inotropic drugs available.

Various drugs may be used to improve the inotropic state of the myocardium (Table 2.6). Those commonly used include digoxin, dopamine, dobu-

TABLE 2.6   Commonly Used Inotropic and Vasoactive Drugs

Drug	Dose (IV)
Digoxin	Loading: 0.75–1.5 mg
	Maintenance: 0.25 mg
Dopamine	Low: 0.5–2.0 µg/kg/min
	Moderate: 2.0–10.0 µg/kg/min
	Large: 10.0–20.0 µg/kg/min
	High: 20.0–50.0 µg/kg/min
Dobutamine	2–10 µg/kg/min
Isoproterenol	1–8 µg/min
Epinephrine	1–8 µg/min
Norepinephrine	1–4 µg/min
Nitroprusside	0.5–10 µg/kg/min
Nitroglycerin	10–20 µg/min

tamine, isoproterenol, epinephrine, and norepinephrine. The goal of inotropic drug therapy is to
improve the position of the ventricular function curve
(via a left shift) so that cardiac output is improved
for each level of cardiac preload. By improving cardiac output, these drugs may be expected to improve
perfusion at the microcirculatory level.

Digoxin is the most commonly used cardiac
glycoside. It should be administered to any patient
in shock that is refractory to volume loading and to
any patient with heart failure in shock. It improves
the force of myocardial contraction and when used
in heart failure causes an augmented cardiac index
and a decreased venous return, promotes diuresis,
and causes a decrease in cardiac size.

Digoxin should be given to any patient in shock refractory to volume loading.

After IV administration, the onset of action of
digoxin is 15–30 minutes. Its peak effect occurs at
1–5 hours. Up to 90% is excreted by the kidneys.
The average digitalizing dose in the adult is 0.75–1.5
mg IV in divided doses over 24 hours. Usually 0.5
mg is given initially by IV, followed by 0.25-mg doses
every 2–12 hours, depending on urgency, until the
total digitalizing dose is given. The usual maintenance dose is 0.25 mg/day. The plasma half-life is
30–36 hours. Digoxin plasma levels can now be
measured by most clinical laboratories, and a maintenance level less than 2.5 mg/ml is usually nontoxic.

How to give digoxin

Dopamine should be the initial sympathomimetic amine used in the treatment of shock refractory to volume loading. It causes a decrease in
peripheral vascular resistance, vasodilation of both
mesenteric and renal vessels, an improved urine output, and an increased cardiac output. It is less arrhythmogenic than the other available catecholamines. The specific hemodynamic response to
dopamine is dose-related. At low doses (0.5–2.0
μg/kg/min), the predominant effects are in the dopaminergic vascular receptors located in the mesenteric and renal vascular beds. Vasodilation in these
areas will improve mesenteric and renal blood flow.
GFR will improve. At moderate doses (2.0–10.0
μg/kg/min) the predominant effects are on the β_1-
adrenergic receptors of the heart, which will increase cardiac contractility and stroke volume. At
larger doses (10.0–20.0 μg/kg/min), the main effects

Dopamine is the sympathomimetic amine of choice.

The effects of dopamine are dose-related.

are on the α-adrenergic vascular receptors, which cause vasoconstriction. At doses higher than 20 μg/kg/min, generalized vasoconstriction will result. Blood pressure will increase but urine output will decrease secondary to renal vasoconstriction. Doses up to 50 μg/kg/min have been used clinically in humans. At levels above 20 μg/kg/min, the α-adrenergic effects dominate and dopamine will act like an infusion of norepinephrine. At high doses, dopamine may actually decrease tissue blood flow and microcirculatory perfusion because of generalized vasoconstriction. This may cause further tissue damage. When using dopamine, therefore, a low rate of infusion (2–5 μg/kg/min) should be selected first. The duration of dopamine action is short and its onset of action is fast, so that the infusion rate can be titrated every few minutes as needed to stabilize the hemodynamic profile.

When using dopamine, a low rate of infusion should be selected first.

Dobutamine

Dobutamine is a newer, potent inotropic agent, which acts mainly on the β-adrenergic receptors. Myocardial contractility and heart rate are increased. Myocardial blood flow may be improved particularly to ischemic areas. Its use in AMI does not increase infarct size. It is less arrhythmogenic than isoproterenol or epinephrine. It has no effect on dopamine receptors. It can, however, have small effects on α-adrenergic receptors, causing vasoconstriction (doses less than 7.5 μg/kg/min), and β_2-adrenergic receptors, causing vasodilation (doses greater than 15 μg/kg/min). The usual starting dose is 2.5–5.0 μg/kg/min. Doses above 20 μg/kg/min should be avoided.

The dose of dobutamine

The use of dobutamine

The clinical role of dobutamine in the treatment of shock is currently unsettled. Since isoproterenol has the side effects of arrhythmogenicity and vasodilation, dobutamine may turn out to be a good substitute for it. In those situations that require both improved myocardial contractility and afterload reduction, the combination of dobutamine and sodium nitroprusside should be considered. This occurs most commonly in the postoperative cardiac patient with low cardiac output.

Isoproterenol

Isoproterenol is a pure β-adrenergic agonist. Its cardiac effects are potent. Both inotropy and heart rate are increased. Vasodilation of mesenteric and skeletal muscle vascular beds may improve blood flow to these areas. Its use in shock is limited, however, because of the significant potential for adverse side effects associated with its use. These include tachycardia, ventricular ectopy, and decreases in blood flow particularly to ischemic areas of the heart. Infarct size may be increased. In addition, it may cause hypotension from vasodilation. The use of isoproterenol is being replaced by dobutamine. If isoproterenol is selected as an inotropic support drug, the dose should be 1–8 μg/min.

Myocardial infarct size may increase with isoproterenol infusion.

Epinephrine is a mixed α, β-adrenergic receptor agonist. Its major effect is on the β_1-receptors, which improve contractility and heart rate. It has no influence on dopamine receptors. At low doses, it has little α-receptor effect but it does stimulate the β_2-receptors. Total peripheral resistance may decrease. At large doses, the α-receptor effects dominate and there may be generalized vasoconstriction. Blood pressure will increase. However, two adverse effects develop: 1) renal vasoconstriction will cause oliguria, and 2) increased afterload (increased total peripheral resistance) will tend to decrease stroke volume and cardiac output. Epinephrine may induce significant tachycardia, and it is very arrhythmogenic. The use of this agent should probably be reserved for the postoperative cardiac surgery patient needing inotropic support and who is refractory to dopamine or dobutamine. The infusion rate should be started at 1 μg/min. Doses up to 8 μg/min may be needed on occasion.

Epinephrine

Adverse effects of epinephrine infusion

Norepinephrine is also a mixed α, β-adrenergic receptor agonist. Its major effect, however, is on the α-receptors. It has little β_1-receptor activity and no β_2-or dopamine receptor activity. Since generalized vasoconstriction results from its use, norepinephrine infusion should be considered only in those hypotensive emergencies refractory to volume loading and inotropic support. The drug should not be used for long periods, since it may enhance tissue ischemia. Tachyphylaxis also results from its prolonged use. The infusion rate should start at 1 μg/min.

Norepinephrine

Norepinephrine should be used only in those hypotensive emergencies refractory to volume loading and inotropic support.

If the circulation is volume-loaded, if the arteriolar resistance is high, and if shock remains refractory to inotropic support, then there is justification for the use of agents that reduce arterial resistance

The use of unloading agents

and thus cardiac afterload. Afterload reduction may improve cardiac performance and the hemodynamic profile.

The use of nitro-
prusside

The α-adrenergic receptor blocking agent phentolamine may be used to decrease arterial resistance but is rarely used clinically nowadays. Afterload reduction is most commoly effected with sodium nitroprusside. This agent has a direct vasodilator effect on both resistance and capacitance vessels. Its onset of action is immediate and its duration of action brief. Its effects are independent of autonomic innervation. An infusion rate of 0.5–10 μg/kg/min may be used. The solution should be protected from light, and solutions older than 4 hours should not be used. Nitroprusside is rapidly metabolized to thiocyanate, blood levels of which can be measured by most clinical laboratories. Levels below 10 mg/100 ml are usually nontoxic. The rate of infusion should be titrated closely to the clinical response. Serial cardiac output measurements will guide clinical responsiveness.

Other vasoactive
agents

Other agents like phenylephrine, methoxamine, mephentermine, metaraminol, angiotensin, and phenoxybenzamine are all potent vasoactive agents that are occasionally used nowadays in the treatment of shock.

The use of calcium

Calcium is needed for normal muscle contraction. When given IV it has a positive inotropic and chronotropic effect on the heart. In patients receiving massive blood transfusions, the level of ionized calcium may become low and hypotension may result. Calcium should be given to those patients acutely transfused 6 units of blood and to those patients in shock from cardiac arrest. Ideally, it should be given through a central venous catheter to prevent skin slough from inadvertent subcutaneous infiltration. Usually 5–10 ml of 10% calcium chloride (500–1000 mg) or 10 ml of 10% calcium gluconate is given over 5–10 minutes. Calcium chloride has more ionizable calcium per volume than does calcium gluconate.

Case Study

A 60-year-old man presents to the emergency room with a several-day history of increasing epigastric pain, nausea, vomiting, and fever for 24 hours. He appears acutely ill and dehydrated. Vital signs reveal a blood pressure of 85/60, pulse 130, respiration 28, and rectal temperature 102.6°F. The upper abdomen is markedly tender with peritoneal signs. Pneumoperitoneum is confirmed on x-ray. A clinical diagnosis of perforated peptic ulcer is made. The following database is obtained: white blood cell count 23,000 with a left shift on differential, hematocrit 49, BUN 90, creatinine 3.2; ABG on room air shows PaO_2 = 65 mm Hg, $PaCO_2$ = 25 mm Hg, and pH 7.28.

A nasogastric tube is passed, a Foley catheter is inserted, a peripheral IV is started with lactated Ringer's solution, and a CVP line is placed. The CVP reads zero with good dynamics. Only 20 ml of urine is obtained initially. The patient is started on broad-spectrum antibiotics and transferred to the surgical intensive care unit for preoperative resuscitation.

Over 30 minutes the patient receives 2 liters of lactated Ringer's. The blood pressure is now 95/70; however, there is still no urine output. The CVP reads 2 cm H_2O. The patient receives a third liter of lactated Ringer's over the next 30 minutes. The blood pressure remains at 95/70, there is still no urine output, and the CVP rises to 12 cm H_2O. At this time a Swan-Ganz catheter and an arterial line are placed. The PCWP measures 8 mm Hg. A fourth liter of lactated Ringer's is given over 30 minutes, and the PCWP increases to 15 mm Hg. The blood pressure increases to 100/70, and the cardiac output is determined to be 3.4 liters/min. The patient is started on dopamine 5 µg/kg/min. The blood pressure increases to 120/70, the cardiac output increases to 4.8 liters/min, and 100 ml of urine is collected over 30 minutes. The patient has now been undergoing resuscitation for 2 hours, and repeat laboratory tests reveal a hematocrit of 40, BUN 60, creatinine 2.5, and an ABG on 40% O_2 by mask shows PaO_2 = 120 mm Hg, $PaCO_2$ = 33 mm Hg, and pH = 7.34. The patient is subsequently brought to surgery, where laparotomy confirms a perforated duodenal ulcer with peritonitis.

The above case illustrates: 1) the importance of accurate monitoring, 2) the principles of fluid volume therapy, and 3) the therapeutic benefit of inotropic drug therapy when volume resuscitation alone fails to improve overall hemodynamic function.

Renal Function

Patients in shock are usually oliguric because of hypotension and hypovolemia. If oliguria persists despite correction of hypovolemia and establishment of normotension, then diuretic therapy is warranted. In this setting, diuretic therapy is both diagnostic of possible acute renal failure (ARF) and therapeutic. The three diuretic agents commonly used are mannitol, furosemide, and ethacrynic acid.

Mannitol is an osmotic diuretic. A test dose of 200 mg/kg (or about 25 g) is infused IV over 5 minutes. The test dose is repeated if there is no incremental increase in the urine output during the next 1–2 hours. If there is failure to respond to this second dose within 3 hours, then more mannitol will not work, ARF should be suspected, and other diuretic agents may be tried. If the urine output improves after the test dose, then a continuous infusion of mannitol can be used. Usually 10–20 ml/h of 10% mannitol (24–48 g/24 h) suffices in maintaining adequate urine volumes. Between 50 and 200 g total may be given over any one 24-hour period.

Some physicians prefer to use loop diuretics instead of mannitol. Furosemide is the most commonly used agent for this purpose. It is a powerful diuretic that inhibits sodium and chloride transport in the ascending limb of Henle's loop. A starting dose of 40 mg is given IV. If there is no response, the dose may be doubled at 30-minute intervals up to 1 g. If there is no response, then ARF exists.

The occasional patient will respond to ethacrynic acid, even if refractory to furosemide. Ethacrynic acid inhibits active chloride reabsorption at the ascending limb of Henle's loop. Fifty to 100 mg may be given IV. If there is no response to ethacrynic acid, then ARF exists.

ARF is an unfortunate occasional complication of shock. Two types exist: 1) low-output ARF (common) and 2) high-output ARF (uncommon). Low-output ARF is characterized by: 1) oliguria, 2) progressive azotemia, 3) decreased glomerular function, 4) decreased renal tubular function, 5) decreased renal concentrating ability, and 6) failure to respond to diuretic challenge after establishment of normovolemia and normotension.

Sometimes high-output ARF may develop, particularly in sepsis. This state is characterized by progressive azotemia despite normal or increased urine volumes. It is one manifestation of ischemic renal injury, although its exact pathophysiology is not understood. Serial measurements of BUN and creatinine levels should be made on all patients in shock to identify those with progressive renal insufficiency despite adequate urine volumes.

Acid-Base Status

Frequent arterial pH measurements should be made. The moribund patient should receive sodium bicarbonate emergently before ABG results are received. Sometimes there may exist an initial alkalosis due to hyperventilation. With severe shock, however, acidemia is the rule. The arterial pH may be below 7.1 on occasion, but more commonly it is in the 7.2–7.35 range due to respiratory compensation. Acidemia depresses myocardial contractility and may decrease the cardiovascular system's responsiveness to catecholamines. It is thus important to correct acidemia so that inotropic drugs will be maximally effective.

> Acidemia depresses cardiac contractility.

> Inotropic drugs may be ineffective at acidemic pHs.

Often the pH will correct when the hemodynamic profile is improved via volume loading. Establishment of normovolemia is therefore important. If the pH is below 7.3, then it is usually necessary to buffer the blood by giving sodium bicarbonate IV while fluid therapy is concurrently being initiated. It is impractical to calculate the amount of bicarbonate needed on the basis of base deficit under these circumstances. If confronted with cardiac arrest or shock in extremis, one or two ampules (50–100 mEq) of sodium bicarbonate may be given safely prior to pH determination. Subsequent therapy can be guided by obtaining frequent (every 8–10 minutes) arterial pH measurements until stable.

> How much bicarbonate to give

Antibiotics

If the patient is in shock and septicemia is suspected, then antibiotics are indicated. Cultures should be obtained as appropriate. Broad-spectrum antibiotics should be selected until culture results become

> If sepsis is suspected, culture the patient and start broad-spectrum antibiotics.

available. The combination of oxacillin (1–2 g IV every 4–6 hours) or ampicillin (1–2 g IV every 4–6 hours) with gentamicin (1–2 mg/kg IV every 8 hours) is commonly used. In patients allergic to penicillin a cephalosporin should be selected in combination with gentamicin. There is about a 10% chance of cross-hypersensitivity reaction to cephalosporins when used in the penicillin-allergic patient. True anaphylaxis is quite rare, and thus their use is very justifiable in the critically ill penicillin-allergic individual.

The commonly used cephalosporins today include cephalothin (1–2 g IV every 4–6 hours), cefazolin (1–2 g IV every 4–8 hours), cefamandole (1–2 g IV every 4–8 hours), cephapirin (1–2 g IV every 4–8 hours), and cefoxitin (1–2 g IV every 4–8 hours). Some physicians prefer cephalosporins over oxacillin or ampicillin initially.

Tobramycin (1–2 mg/kg IV every 8 hours) may be used instead of gentamicin. This newer aminoglycoside antibiotic has recently been shown to be less nephrotoxic than gentamicin. If the possibility of anaerobic septicemia exists, for example, in intra-abdominal sepsis or septic abortion, then clindamycin (300–600 mg IV every 6 hours) or metronidazole (7.5 mg/kg IV every 6 hours) should be added to the above two-drug regimen. Alternatively, chloramphenicol (50 mg/kg/day in four divided doses or 0.5–1.0 g IV every 6 hours) may be combined with oxacillin until culture results return.

Steroids

Steroids in pharmacologic doses should be given in septic shock or when adrenal insufficiency is suspected.

There is a large literature, much of it controversial, on the use of corticosteroids in the treatment of shock. In septic shock pharmacologic doses of steroids seem beneficial. However, their use in hemorrhagic or cardiogenic shock is of unproven value at present. It is known from clinical studies in humans that a bolus IV dose of 30 mg/kg methylprednisolone (about 2 g in the adult) or its equivalent dose improves survival in septic shock. This dose may be repeated as needed at 4-hour intervals for 24–48 hours. The incidence of serious adverse reactions from steroid use, such as acute gastrointestinal hemorrhage, increases when multiple doses are required.

How steroids work in sepsis is not known. Their effects are multiple and include: 1) stabilization of lysosomal membranes in the lung, pancreas, liver, and kidneys; 2) stabilization of vascular membranes in the lung and intestine; 3) improved cardiac contractility; 4) improved oxygen consumption; 5) decreased vascular resistance in the lung, intestine, and kidneys; and 6) enhancement of lactic acid metabolism. Obviously, steroids should be given to any patient in shock suspected of adrenal insufficiency. This is often difficult to determine acutely, and thus many physicians use steroids empirically to protect against this possibility.

The effects of steroids

Electrolyte Status

Serum electrolytes should be measured and disturbances corrected as indicated. This is particularly true for serum potassium abnormalities.

Coagulation Status

If the PT is elevated greater than 2 seconds above normal, corrective therapy with vitamin K and FFP should begin. Platelet transfusions are indicated for the bleeding patient with a platelet count less than 50,000. If a consumptive DIC syndrome is suspected, the diagnosis should be confirmed by measuring fibrin split products and fibrinogen levels. Treatment of the DIC syndrome mainly involves controlling the inciting event. Heparin therapy is rarely indicated in this syndrome and has fallen out of vogue.

Use platelet transfusion in the bleeding patient with platelet count less than 50,000.

Temperature Status

The patient should be made normothermic as soon as feasible. Acetaminophen (10–20 grains) may be administered as a rectal suppository every 4 hours as needed. If this drug is not successful in lowering body temperature, then alcohol sponge baths and a cooling blanket should be used. Conversely, hypothermia should be corrected with a heating blanket as needed.

Reestablish normothermia.

Prevention of Gastrointestinal Bleeding

Use antacids liberally.

Acute gastritis and gastroduodenal erosion and ulceration are an unfortunate complication of shock. The prophylactic use of antacid agents is warranted in these stressed patients. The H_2 receptor antagonist cimetidine may be used in doses up to 300 mg IV every 4 hours. Antacids (30–120 ml/h via mouth or nasogastric tube) will suffice. There is recent clincial evidence supporting the view that antacids are better than cimetidine in the prophylaxis against stress ulceration. Gastric pH should be titrated to above 4.0 to prevent pepsinogen conversion to pepsin. This may be accomplished on an hourly basis using a nasogastric tube and pH paper at the bedside. Of interest is a recent study which showed that cimetidine alone fails to raise the gastric pH above 4.0 in 25% of critically ill patients.

Titrate gastric pH to above pH 4.

Nutrition

The patient resuscitated from shock is maximally stressed and has a marked increase in metabolic demands. Attention should eventually be directed at alimentation. The oral route is preferred if feasible. If the gastrointestinal tract is intact but the patient is unable to eat, then continuous tube feedings can be instituted using a liquid formula diet. If it can be accurately estimated that the patient will be taking oral alimentation within a week of the shock insult, then peripheral hyperalimentation with amino acid solutions and lipid may be used in the interim. If the duration of starvation is estimated to be longer than that, then central hyperalimentation using hypertonic glucose and amino acids should be started promptly. This may also be supplemented by lipid extract IV to supply lipid calories and essential free fatty acids (10–20% Intralipid).

If the patient will not be eating for 5 days after the shock insult, then alimentation is indicated early.

Annotated Bibliography

Baue AE. Recent developments in the study and treatment of shock. Surg Gynecol Obstet 127:849–878, 1968.

A detailed review article about shock with an extensive list of references.

Baue AE. Metabolic abnormalities of shock. Surg Clin North Am 56:1059–1071, 1976.
A succinct review of the metabolic alterations in shock.

Chaudry IH, Clemens MG, Baue AE. Alterations in cell function with ischemia and shock and their correction. Arch Surg 116:1309–1317, 1981.
A current model of cellular dysfunction in shock is presented.

Ledingham EM (ed). Shock. Clinical and Experimental Aspects. American Elsevier, New York, 1976.
A detailed account of many of the pathophysiologic abnormalities in shock.

McGovern VJ. Shock. Pathol Annu 6:279–298, 1971.
A detailed review of the pathology of organs in shock.

Moore FD. The effects of hemorrhage on body composition. N Engl J Med 273:567–577, 1965.
A classic paper describing the phenomenon of plasma refill following hemorrhage.

Shires GT, Carrico CJ, Canizaro PC. Shock. W. B. Saunders, Philadelphia, 1973.
An excellent monograph on the diagnosis and treatment of shock.

Swan HJC, Ganz W. Use of balloon flotation catheters in critically ill patients. Surg Clin North Am 55:501–520, 1975.
How to use Swan-Ganz catheters in clinical practice.

Additional Bibliography

Alko A, Jaattela A, Lahdensuu M, et al. Catecholamines in shock. Ann Clin Res 9:157–163, 1977.

Amato TJ, Rheinlander HF, Cleveland RJ. Post-traumatic adult respiratory distress syndrome. Orthop Clin North Am 9:693–713, 1978.

Austen WG, Buckley MJ. Treatment of various forms of surgical shock. Prog Cardiovasc Dis 10:97–116, 1967.

Baue AE. The energy crisis in surgical patients. Arch Surg 109:349–350, 1974

Baue AE, Wurth MA, Chaudry IH, et al. Impairment of cell membrane transport during shock and after treatment. Ann Surg 178:412–422, 1973.

Baue AE, Chaudry IH, Wurth MA, et al. Cellular alterations with shock and ischemia. Angiology 25:41–42, 1974.

Baxter CR. Shock and metabolism. Surg Gynecol Obstet 142:216–219, 1976.

Berk JL. Monitoring the patient in shock. Surg Clin North Am 55:713–720, 1975.

Buchbinder N, Ganz W. Hemodynamic monitoring. Anesthesia 45:146–155, 1976.

Chaudry IH, Sayeed MM, Baue AE. Depletion and restoration of tissue ATP in hemorrhagic shock. Arch Surg 108:208–211, 1974.

Clauss RH, Ray TF III. Pharmacologic assistance to the failing circulation. Surg Gynecol Obstet 126:611–631,1968.

Cowley RA, Mergner WJ. Fisher RS, et al. The subcellular pathology of shock in trauma patients: Studies using the immediate autopsy. Am Surg 45:255–269, 1979.

Cunningham JW, Shires GT, Wagner Y. Cellular transport defects in hemorrhagic shock. Surgery 70:215–222, 1971.

Egdahl RH, Meguid MM, Aun F. The importance of the endocrine and metabolic responses to shock and trauma. Crit Care Med 5:257–263, 1977.

Fritz SD. Energy metabolism in shock. Heart Lung 4:615–618, 1975.

Garcia-Barreno P, Balibrea JL. Metabolic response in shock. Surg Gynecol Obstet 146:182–189, 1978.

Garcia-Barreno P, Balibrea JL, Aparicio P. Blood coagulation changes in shock. Surg Gynecol Obstet 147:6–12, 1978.

Gelin L. Reaction of the body as a whole to injury. J. Trauma 10:932–939, 1970.

Haljamae H, Amundson B, Bagge U, et al. Pathophysiology of shock. Pathol Res Pract 165:200–211, 1979.

Hardaway RM III. Monitoring of the patient in a state of shock. Surg Gynecol Obstet 148:339–345, 1979.

Herman CM. Advances and newer concepts in shock—1972. Surg Annu 4:1–49, 1972.

Hershey SG (ed). Shock. Little, Brown, Boston, 1964.

Jakschik BA, Marshall GR, Kourik JL, et al. Profile of

circulating vasoactive substances in hemorrhagic shock and their pharmacologic manipulation. J Clin Invest 54:842–852, 1974.

Latts JR, Goldberg LI. Dopamine in the management of shock. Drug Therapy, pp 25–30, January 1979.

Levy MN. The cardiovascular physiology of the critically ill patinet. Surg Clin North Am 55:483–499, 1975.

Long DM Jr, Rose AL, Malone LVW, et al. Blood rheology in trauma patients. Surg Clin North Am 52:19–30, 1972.

MacLean LD, Duff JH, Scott HM, et al. Treatment of shock in man based on hemodynamic diagnosis. Surg Gynecol Obstet 120:1–16, 1965.

McConn R. The oxyhemoglobin dissociation curve in acute disease. Surg Clin North Am 55:627–658, 1975.

Nickerson M. Vascular adjustments during the development of shock. Can Med Assoc J 103:853–859, 1970.

O'Donnel TF Jr, Belkin SC. The pathophysiology, monitoring and treatment of shock. Orthop Clin North Am 9:589–610, 1978.

Plachetka JR. Sympathomimetic pharmacology. Crit Care Q 2:27–35, 1980.

Pontoppidau H, Geffin B, Lowenstein E. Acute respiratory failure in the adult. N Engl J Med 287:690–698, 1972.

Reichgott MJ, Melmon KL. Should corticosteroids be used in shock? Med Clin North Am 57:1211–1223, 1973.

Riede V, Sandritter W, Mittermayer C. Circulatory shock: A review. Pathology 13:299–311, 1981.

Sabiston DC Jr (ed). Davis-Christopher Textbook of Surgery. W. B. Saunders, Philadelphia, 1981.

Schumer W. Shock and its effect on the cell. JAMA 205:75–79, 1968.

Schumer W. Metabolic aspects of shock. Surg Annu 6:1–16, 1974.

Schumer W. Metabolism during shock and sepsis. Heart Lung 5:416–421, 1976.

Schumer W, Kukral JC. Metabolism of shock. Surgery 63:630–636, 1968.

Shah M, Browner BD, Dutton RE, et al. Cardiac output and pulmonary wedge pressure. Arch Surg 112:1161–1164, 1977.

Shires GT, Cunningham JW, Baker CRF, et al. Alterations in cellular membrane function during hemorrhagic shock in primates. Ann Surg 176:288–295, 1972.

Shoemaker WC. Tissue perfusion defects in shock and trauma states. Surg Gynecol Obstet 137:980–986, 1973.

Shoemaker WC. Pathobiology of death: Structural and functional interactions in shock syndromes. Pathobiol Annu 6:365–407, 1976.

Sugerman JH, Roger RM, Miller LD. Positive end-expiratory pressure (PEEP): Indications and physiologic considerations. Chest 62:865–945, 1972.

Walt AJ, Wilson RF. The treatment of shock. Adv Surg 9:1–39, 1975.

Wayne KS. Positive end-expiratory pressure (PEEP) ventilation. JAMA 236:1394–1396, 1976.

Weil MH, Shubin H, Carlson R. Treatment of circulatory shock. JAMA 231:1280–1286, 1975.

Hemorrhagic Shock and Trauma

3

Overview

Hemorrhagic shock is that shock syndrome caused by a significant decrease in blood volume due to bleeding. Trauma is a major cause. Usually at least 20% of the total blood volume must be lost acutely in the adult to induce shock. The body responds to this volume loss in three major ways: 1) the sympathetic nervous system is activated; 2) the endocrine system is activated with secretion of epinephrine, ADH, and aldosterone; and 3) there are fluid shifts via plasma refill. The therapy of hemorrhagic shock involves: 1) controlling the hemorrhage; 2) reestablishing normovolemia using blood and Ringer's lactate solution; and 3) improving cardiac performance using inotropic agents, sodium bicarbonate, and calcium chloride.

Definition

Hemorrhagic shock can be defined as that shock syndrome caused by a significant decrease in blood volume due to bleeding. Hypovolemic shock is that shock syndrome which results from any condition that significantly decreases circulatory volume, whether whole blood volume, plasma volume, or extracellular, extravascular fluid volume.

Etiology

All those conditions that cause significant bleeding may cause hemorrhagic shock. These commonly include: 1) traumatic hemorrhage; 2) gastrointestinal hemorrhage; 3) operative hemorrhage; 4) aneurysm

Common causes of hemorrhagic shock

87

rupture; 5) obstetrical hemorrhage; and 6) massive hemoptysis.

The causes of hypovolemic shock due to loss of plasma volume or extracellular, extravascular fluid volume include: 1) thermal trauma; 2) peritonitis; 3) pancreatitis; 4) enterocolitis; 5) bowel obstruction; 6) mesenteric ischemia or thrombosis; and 7) diabetes mellitus or insipidus.

In the United States trauma is the third most common cause of death (after atherosclerosis and cancer) and is the leading cause of death among those less than 45 years old. In 1980 trauma claimed 164,000 lives. The most common cause of traumatic death is motor vehicle accidents. Each year there are about 26 million driver accidents, which cause about 50,000 deaths. In addition, the homicide rate tripled in the 20-year period 1960–1980. In 1980 there were 27,800 murders. The overall cost to society of this great volume of traumatic injury has been estimated to be about 75 million dollars per day.

Traumatic injuries can be classified as either blunt or penetrating, depending upon the mechanism of the injury. In penetrating abdominal trauma the small bowel is the most frequently injured organ (Table 3.1). In blunt abdominal trauma the spleen is the most commonly injured organ (Table 3.2). In

Common causes of decreased plasma and extracellular fluid volume

The total financial burden to society of traumatic injury is about 75 million dollars per day.

TABLE 3.1 Incidence of Organ Injury in Penetrating Abdominal Trauma

Organ	Percentage
Small bowel	30%
Mesentery, omentum	18
Liver	16
Colon	9
Diaphragm	8
Stomach	7
Spleen	6
Kidney	5
Major blood vessel	4
Pancreas	3
Duodenum	2
Bladder	1
Ureter	1
Biliary	1

Reprinted with permission from Blaisdell FW, Trunkey DD. *Abdominal Trauma.* Thieme-Stratton, New York, 1982, p 11.

TABLE 3.2   Incidence of Organ Injury in Blunt Abdominal Trauma

Organ	Percentage
Spleen	25%
Liver	15
Retroperitoneal hematoma	13
Kidney	12
Small bowel	9
Bladder	6
Mesentery	5
Large bowel	4
Pancreas	3
Urethra	2
Diaphragm	2
Major blood vessel	2
Stomach	1
Duodenum	1

Reprinted with permission from Blaisdell FW, Trunkey DD. *Abdominal Trauma*. Thieme-Stratton, New York, 1982, p 13.

general, gunshot wounds of the abdomen have a greater than 90% chance of causing visceral injury, whereas abdominal stab wounds have only about a 40% chance of causing visceral injury.

Diagnosis

The diagnosis of hemorrhagic shock is usually straightforward, except in blunt abdominal trauma. Much can be learned from the antecedent history. For example, the patient may relate a history of hematemesis or melanotic stools. This information may expedite the diagnosis and workup.

All trauma victims in shock should be suspected of having a significant hemorrhagic injury. During and after initial resuscitative efforts, a prompt search for the source of bleeding must be accomplished. In blunt abdominal trauma this may involve the use of diagnostic peritoneal lavage.

All trauma victims in shock should be suspected of having hemorrhagic injury.

Clinical Findings

The clinical findings in hemorrhagic shock are due to a combination of diminished blood volume and activation of both the sympathetic nervous system

The clinical findings depend on the amount of blood loss.

and the neuroendocrine (sympathoadrenal) axis. With minimal blood loss (less than 15% total blood volume) the patient may appear entirely normal. Compensatory vasoconstriction of arteriolar resistance vessels will maintain blood pressure, and compensatory venoconstriction of venous capacitance vessels will augment effective blood volume and cardiac preload.

With moderate blood loss (20–30% total blood volume) there is usually sinus tachycardia and postural hypotension. The respiratory rate increases. The skin is moist and cool. There may be accompanying pallor. The skin capillary refill test (blanching test) is prolonged above the normal 1.5 seconds. The patient may appear anxious or apprehensive. Urine output decreases as blood flow is redistributed to more vital organs, especially the heart and the brain. The central venous pressure (CVP) is low.

With severe hemorrhage (greater than 30% total blood volume) there is sustained hypotension and sinus tachycardia. Respirations may become agonal. The skin is cold. There may be cyanosis with cutaneous mottling. The patient may show lethargy, stupor, or coma. Urine output is minimal. The CVP approaches zero.

From the above, it is clear that the signs and symptoms of hemorrhage depend on the magnitude of the hemorrhagic insult. The body is able to compensate totally for decreases of less than 15% of the blood volume. In general, at least 20–25% of the blood volume must be acutely lost in order for the hemorrhagic shock syndrome to develop. With this degree of blood loss the endogenous homeostatic mechanisms cannot compensate fully and shock may result.

The body can usually compensate for loss of 15% of blood volume.

Any patient in shock from gastrointestinal bleeding, trauma, obstetrical hemorrhage, etc., can be assumed to have lost 20–25% of his or her total blood volume. This means that at least 1000 ml of whole blood has been lost acutely in the adult. With the acute loss of 30% or more of the blood volume, almost all patients will present in shock. It should be noted that with an acute loss of 20% of the blood volume there is much individual patient variation in the extent of the signs and symptoms of ongoing

Any patient in hemorrhagic shock has lost at least 20% of blood volume.

hemorrhage. What may be a fairly well tolerated insult for the young adult may be a lethal injury for
the geriatric patient.

The signs of intra-abdominal injury and hemorrhage after blunt abdominal trauma may be subtle.
It is possible for life-threatening intra-abdominal
hemorrhage to occur without any change in abdominal girth. This is so because the main dimensional
change with intraperitoneal bleeding is in a vertical
direction, with displacement of the diaphragm. The
abdominal wall may appear normal and without
contusion or ecchymosis. Most awake patients, however, with hemoperitoneum after blunt trauma will
have abdominal tenderness on exam.

The clinical findings of intra-abdominal injury following abdominal trauma may be subtle.

Peritoneal Lavage

Diagnostic peritoneal lavage is an extremely useful
method of evaluating the presence of significant
intra-abdominal injury following blunt trauma. Strict
guidelines for which patients should be lavaged following trauma have not been established. The de-
cision to lavage and the actual performance of the
procedure should be done by the general surgeon
who has ultimate responsibility for the care of the
trauma victim. One must, therefore, consult the general surgeon promptly in these situations.

In general the indications for lavage after blunt
abdominal trauma include unstable vital signs, abdominal tenderness, falling hematocrit, and index of
clinical suspicion as, for example, in multiple trauma
with associated head injury. Any patient with head
trauma, altered mental status, and shock following
traumatic injury must be assumed to be bleeding in-
traperitoneally until proven otherwise. Peritoneal lavage is a direct and accurate way to confirm the diagnosis in these circumstances.

The indications for diagnostic peritoneal lavage

There are three ways to perform peritoneal lavage. These include: 1) the Lazarus-Nelson needle
and stylet technique; 2) the dialysis catheter-trocar
technique; and 3) the open lavage technique.

How to perform peritoneal lavage

The Lazarus-Nelson technique is currently
popular. A Foley catheter and a nasogastric tube must
be passed prior to the procedure. The infraumbilical

The Lazarus-Nelson technique

area is prepped and draped. Lidocaine 1% with epinephrine is used as local anesthesia. With a #11 blade a small skin incision is executed in the midline down to the linea alba, which is incised for about 2 mm. An 18-gauge needle is then inserted via this incision through the fascia and peritoneum. A guide wire is then inserted through this needle and directed toward the pelvis. The needle is removed and a 9 French Teflon catheter is placed over the guide wire, directed toward the pelvis, and the wire is removed.

The dialysis catheter-trocar technique

The dialysis catheter-trocar technique is performed as follows. A Foley catheter and a nasogastric tube must be passed prior to this procedure. The infraumbilical area is shaved, prepped, and draped. Lidocaine 1% with epinephrine is used for local anesthesia. A midline incision is executed starting about 1 cm inferior to the umbilicus and is extended for about 2 cm in length. Dissection is carried down to the midline fascia, which is incised for about a 3-mm distance. The skin, subcutaneous fat, and fascia are elevated using a towel clip, and a dialysis catheter with trocar is then inserted into the peritoneal cavity. The trocar is removed as the catheter is directed toward the pelvis.

The open lavage technique

The open lavage technique is performed as follows. Again, a Foley catheter and a nasogastric tube must be passed. The infraumbilical area is shaved, prepped, and draped. Lidocaine 1% with epinephrine is used for local anesthesia. A midline incision is executed about 1 cm inferior to the umbilicus and is extended for about 2 cm. Dissection under direct vision is continued through subcutaneous tissue and fascia, and the peritoneum is opened. A dialysis catheter may then be placed directly into the abdomen and directed toward the pelvis.

If gross blood returns, then the tap is positive and no lavage is necessary. If the tap fails to return blood, then 1 liter of lactated Ringer's or normal saline (20 ml/kg in children) is instilled into the peritoneal cavity. The fluid is then withdrawn by placing the bottle of saline on the floor beneath the patient. If bloody fluid returns, the test is considered positive.

Parameters to measure in the lavage fluid

If one cannot read newsprint through the blood-tinged fluid, then the test is also considered positive.

TABLE 3.3   Positive Criteria in Peritoneal Lavage in Blunt Abdominal Trauma

Gross blood
Inability to read newsprint through bloody lavage fluid
$>$100,000 RBC/mm^3 of lavage fluid
$>$500 WBC/mm^3 of lavage fluid
$>$175 amylase units/100 ml of lavage fluid
Bile, bacteria, or intestinal contents on microscopic exam of
   lavage fluid.

RBC, red blood cells; WBC, white blood cells.

If the returning fluid is slightly pink (equivocal), the following data obtained on the lavage fluid are also indicative of a positive lavage: greater than 100,000 red blood cells per mm^3; more than 500 white blood cells per mm^3; an amylase value of greater than 175 units per 100 ml; or bile, intestinal contents, or bacteria in the fluid (Table 3.3).

A positive lavage is 97% accurate in diagnosing significant intra-abdominal injury. This means that only about 3% of patients with positive lavage will have a negative exploratory laparotomy. Likewise, the accuracy of a negative lavage is over 98%. Fewer than 2% of the patients with a negative lavage will have a positive exploratory laparotomy. The complication rate of peritoneal lavage is under 2%.

Accuracy of lavage

A few additional points are warranted. First, in young children the open technique is preferred. Some surgeons prefer this method routinely in adults as well. Second, if the patient has undergone previous abdominal surgery and may have adhesions to the anterior abdominal wall, then the open technique is preferred. Third, if the patient has a signficant pelvic fracture, there is the potential for extension of a retroperitoneal hematoma up the anterior abdominal wall. This may lead to a false positive lavage if done in the infraumbilical location using one of the closed techniques. In this instance an open lavage should be performed in the midline in a supraumbilical location. Fourth, in the multiple trauma victim with an equivocal lavage it may well be wise to leave the lavage catheter in place for a few hours so that the patient can be relavaged without the added risk of catheter reinsertion.

Some finer points about peritoneal lavage

▦ Pathophysiology

The pathophysiology of hemorrhagic shock involves a marked reduction in whole blood volume due to bleeding. Blood volume is one of the major determinants of cardiac preload. Hemorrhage causes a decrease in blood volume and subsequently in cardiac preload. The systemic function curve shifts down and to the left. This results in a new circulatory equilibrium point (point B in Figure 3.1). Both preload and cardiac output decrease.

Hemorrhage causes a leftward shift in the systemic function curve.

There are three major homeostatic mechanisms that counteract the acute effects of hemorrhage on circulatory performance. These include: 1) hemodynamic adjustments, 2) hormonal adjustments, and 3) volume adjustments. The function of these adjustments is to increase blood volume, increase cardiac output, and increase blood pressure.

There are three homeostatic mechanisms activated in hypovolemic shock.

The hemodynamic adjustments involve the activation of the sympathetic nervous system. This causes: 1) vasoconstiction of arteriolar resistance vessels, 2) venoconstriction of venous capacitance vessels, 3) increased cardiac contractility and heart rate, and 4) redistribution of blood flow away from skin, muscle, kidney, and mesentery to the most vital organs, the heart and the brain.

Hemodynamic adjustments following blood loss

The hormonal adjustments in shock involve the activation of the neuroendocrine axis. Epinephrine secreted by the adrenal medulla causes vasoconstriction, increased cardiac contractility, and increased heart rate. Water and salt are conserved by the actions of aldosterone and ADH on the nephron.

Hormonal adjustments following blood loss

Further volume adjustments involve the process of plasma refill. Interstitial fluid moves rapidly into the intravascular space. The magnitude of plasma refill depends on the severity of hypovolemia. With severe hemorrhage, plasma refill rates may approach 1000 ml in the first hour. This process accounts for the low hematocrits obtained soon after major hemorrhage. Plasma refill is complete at about 40 hours posthemorrhage. The volume of new plasma added to the vascular space equals the volume of shed whole blood.

Volume adjustments following blood loss

The above-described homeostatic mechanisms affect the cardiac, the vascular, and the fluid volume components of the circulation. The homeostatic response to hemorrhagic shock thus involves an integration of the cardiac system with the vascular system. This may be viewed graphically (Figure 3.1). As mentioned earlier, a decrease in blood volume will shift the systemic function curve to the left. This moves the circulatory equilibrium point from point A to point B. Homeostatic improvements in blood volume (via venoconstriction, ADH, aldosterone, and plasma refill) will shift the systemic function curve back in a rightward direction. Improved cardiac performance (via improved contractility and heart rate) will shift the cardiac function curve to the left. The

The homeostatic response in hemorrhagic shock involves adjustments in both the cardiac and systemic function curves.

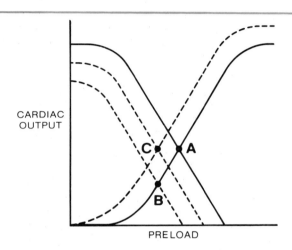

CARDIAC
OUTPUT

PRELOAD

FIGURE 3.1 Hemorrhagic shock is due to an acute decrease in whole blood volume. This causes the systemic function curve to shift downward and to the left. A new equilibrium point (B) is reached, representing a decrease in cardiac output. The body responds by: 1) increasing blood volume (via venoconstriction, plasma refill, ADH, and aldosterone) and 2) improving cardiac performance (via improved contractility and heart rate). These mechanisms shift the systemic function curve upward and to the right and shift the ventricular function curve upward and to the left. The new, compensated equilibrium point (C) represents an improved hemodynamic state over point B. Adapted with permission from Kelman GR. Applied Cardiovascular Physiology. Butterworths, Woburn MA, 1977, p 125.

resulting new equilibrium, point C, represents an improved hemodynamic state over point B in that for each level of cardiac preload there is improved cardiac output.

If the blood volume deficit is small, the normal homeostatic mechanisms may suffice in preserving circulatory function. If the blood volume deficit is severe, however, these mechanisms may fail to compensate adequately, and the patient may die unless the appropriate therapeutic intervention is undertaken rapidly.

Treatment

Treatment includes reestablishing normovolemia and improving cardiac performance.

Treating hypovolemic shock involves: 1) reestablishing normovolemia and 2) improving cardiac performance. These two functions are interrelated. Improving the volume status will often improve the cardiac status, due to the influence of preload on stroke volume. The objective of volume loading in hypovolemic states, therefore, is to maximize ventricular preload. Volume is administered until the plateau, horizontal phase of the cardiac function curve is attained. This occurs in most adults at a CVP of 12–15 cm H_2O or a mean pulmonary capillary wedge pressure (PCWP) of 15–18 mm Hg. Above these levels there is little gain in cardiac output. Indeed, if these levels are indiscriminately surpassed, iatrogenic heart failure and pulmonary edema may result. If shock remains refractory to volume loading, attention must be directed at improving cardiac contractility and vascular tone.

General Measures

As in any resuscitative effort, control of the airway and adequate ventilation are the first objectives (Table 3.4). Once established, attention can then be directed at the circulation.

In hemorrhagic shock, several large bore 14- or 16-gauge Jelco intracatheters should be placed for intravenous access. The upper extremities are preferred in trauma victims. A CVP catheter should be

TABLE 3.4   Priorities in Treatment of Hemorrhagic Shock

1) Secure airway
2) Control external bleeding sites
3) Insert two large-bore IVs
4) Start crystalloid solution
5) Send baseline blood work
6) Insert Foley catheter
7) Insert CVP line
8) Elevate legs
9) Use the MAST suit
10) Splint fractures
11) Obtain chest x-ray
12) Obtain EKG
13) Insert nasogastric tube, if indicated
14) Start antibiotics, if indicated

inserted. A Foley catheter should next be inserted into the bladder, unless there is obvious urethral injury. Urethral disruption in the trauma victim can sometimes be ascertained by noting blood at the urethral meatus or by noting a floating prostate gland on digital rectal exam. If these are found, or if the pubic bone is fractured, a retrograde urethrogram should be performed prior to Foley catheterization.

In abdominal trauma with shock, a nasogastric tube should be placed in the stomach, unless there is an associated basilar skull fracture. Rarely a nasogastric tube may be passed through a basilar skull fracture into the brain with obvious tragic results. The patient's legs should be elevated, but the Trendelenburg position is avoided.

All sites of external bleeding are controlled using direct digital pressure. Blind clamping and tourniquet application should be avoided.

In hemorrhagic shock due to trauma, military antishock trousers (MAST suit) should be applied. Since 1973 the MAST suit has been used in the initial treatment of the hypotensive civilian trauma victim. Nowadays it is routine for paramedic personnel to apply this garment at the scene. The MAST suit works mainly by increasing total peripheral vascular resistance and thus blood pressure rather than by significantly increasing venous return and cardiac preload and stroke volume. The MAST suit can be inflated to a maximum pressure of 104 mm Hg. Usually about 40 mm Hg is adequate to reverse most

Use of the MAST suit

cases of trauma-induced hypotension. If inflation of the MAST suit is required to attain hemodynamic stability, then the suit should remain inflated while the initial hospital diagnostic workup is undertaken and the patient is transported to the operating room.

Blood samples are drawn for type and cross-match, complete blood count, blood chemistries (glucose, BUN, electrolytes, amylase), coagulation profile (PT, PTT, platelet count), and arterial blood gas analysis. An EKG is obtained, as is a portable chest x-ray.

Volume Therapy

Crystalloid Solutions   W. Arbuthnot Lane of Great Britain about 90 years ago was the first to use normal saline infusion in the treatment of hemorrhagic shock. Much has been written about fluid resuscitation in shock since that time. Apart from sanguineous solutions (whole blood, packed red blood cells) there are two major types of asanguineous solutions available: 1) crystalloid solutions (Ringer's lactate, normal saline) and 2) colloid solutions (albumin, fresh frozen plasma [FFP], plasma protein fraction [PPF], dextran).

Types of asanguineous solutions

Shires and colleagues showed in the early 1960s that there is a decrease in the extracellular fluid compartment, as measured by tagged radiosulfate, during hemorrhage. This involves movement of fluid from the interstitial space to the intravascular space. Crystalloid solutions diffuse freely into the interstitial space. Their use in hemorrhagic shock has a good theoretical basis. Crystalloids can restore both the intravascular volume deficit and the extracellular (interstitial) fluid compartment deficit.

In hemorrhagic shock there is an extracellular, interstitial compartment deficit. Crystalloids can restore this space and also intravascular volume.

Initial crystalloid fluid therapy

In the initial management of hemorrhagic shock, therefore, 1–2 liters of Ringer's lactate is administered intravenously in about 15 minutes. This has three major functions: 1) it allows time for proper crossmatching of type-specific blood, 2) it serves as an indicator of continuing hemorrhage, and 3) it helps to replenish the fluid losses of the intravascular and interstitial fluid compartments. If the hemodynamic profile becomes unstable or remains unstable after this fluid challenge, then there is probably continuing hemorrhage.

Ringer's lactate has certain advantages over normal saline. The electrolyte composition of Ringer's lactate solution more closely approximates that of plasma. Normal saline has a lower pH (5.0) than Ringer's lactate (6.5). Fifty percent of the 28 mEq per liter of lactate in Ringer's lactate is in the metabolically active levorotatory form. Thus there are 14 mEq L-lactate per liter available for conversion to bicarbonate buffer by the liver. Although the metabolism of lactate to bicarbonate by the liver during shock is not totally efficient, it does supply some buffering advantage.

Reasons for using Ringer's lactate as initial volume therapy in hemorrhagic shock

The argument that Ringer's lactate infusion during hemorrhagic shock may augment the metabolic lactic acidemia of shock is unfounded. Clinical studies from Vietnam have shown that there is no difference in either arterial lactate levels or acid-base status between patients resuscitated with Ringer's lactate plus blood and those with normal saline plus blood. By improving overall circulatory function and tissue perfusion, Ringer's lactate solution actually helps correct the lactic acidemia of shock. In addition, clinical studies have shown that the use of crystalloid solution significantly diminishes blood transfusion requirements.

Blood Products In the trauma victim, fresh whole blood should ideally be used. This is rarely available and thus component therapy with packed red blood cells, FFP, and platelets is currently standard.

Component therapy is standard practice.

The hematocrit should be maintained at between 30 and 35. At this level the rheologic properties of blood are actually improved due to decreased blood viscosity. In addition, raising the hematocrit above these levels causes little gain in extra oxygen-carrying capacity of blood.

Dilution of clotting factors and platelets during massive transfusion (>6 units of blood) can cause a dilutional coagulopathy and bleeding. This makes the surgeon's job all the more difficult. In general, about 1 unit of FFP should be given for each 4–5 units of packed red blood cells. Platelet counts should be measured periodically, and as a guide about 10 units of prepared platelets should be given for each 8 units of packed red blood cells.

In general, 1 unit of FFP should be given for each 4–5 units of blood and 10 units of platelets should be given for each 8 units of blood.

Colloid Products There is little place for the use of colloid solutions in the treatment of ongoing

Albumin should not
be used in hemor-
rhagic shock.

hemorrhagic shock. The best results are obtained by
using blood and Ringer's lactate solution.

The experience from Vietnam showed that those
patients resuscitated with albumin in saline required
about twice as much blood and put out half as much
urine compared to those resuscitated with crystalloid solutions and blood. The clinical impression
was that the albumin-in-saline patients did worse.

It is known that plasma colloid osmotic pressure decreases with crystalloid resuscitation in hemorrhagic shock. There is no clear evidence, however,
that the infusion of crystalloids causes pulmonary
dysfunction by lowering the colloid osmotic pressure. Indeed, there are some data to suggest that crystalloid resuscitation actually corrects the interstitial
edema of pulmonary tissue after hemorrhagic shock,
whereas colloid resuscitation does not.

In the Vietnam studies, those patients receiving
albumin in saline did not have higher protein or albumin levels, despite receiving on the average 250
g of albumin. Albumin should not be used in the
initial resuscitation of hemorrhagic shock for the following reasons: 1) it offers no advantages over crystalloid solutions, 2) patients may actually do worse
clinically, and 3) it is expensive.

Colloid therapy can be
used selectively in
hypovolemic states.

Colloid therapy can be used selectively in hypovolemic states or nonhemorrhagic hypovolemic
shock. Its use should be limited to the following:
1) the nonhemorrhaging patient with hematocrit above
35; 2) the patient who requires strict salt restriction,
such as the cirrhotic; and 3) the hypoproteinemic
patient.

There are five major colloid solutions available
for clinical use: 1) FFP, 2) albumin, 3) PPF (Plasmanate, Plasmatein), 4) dextran, and 5) hetastarch.

FFP is most commonly used and is readily
available. It carries a hepatitis risk, however.

Normal human serum albumin is at least 96%
pure albumin. It is derived from blood plasma. There
have been no cases of hepatitis associated with its
use. It is available as either a 5% or a 25% solution
in saline. The 5% solution is osmotically equivalent
to its volume of plasma, whereas the 25% solution
is osmotically equivalent to five times its volume of
plasma.

PPF, also derived from blood plasma, is 83–90%
pure albumin. It is available as a 5% solution. Like

normal human serum albumin, there have been no cases of hepatitis associated with its use.

Dextran is a glucose polymer that is available as either dextran 40 (low molecular weight) or dextran 70 (high molecular weight). Like albumin, it acts as a plasma colloid to support blood volume. Dextran 40 increases plasma volume by about twice the volume administered, whereas dextran 70 increases plasma volume only slightly. Dextran can no longer be recommended as a plasma expander for the following reasons: 1) there is a risk of anaphylaxis with its use, 2) there is an increased bleeding tendency with its use as a result of decreased platelet adhesiveness, 3) dextran interferes with blood typing and crossmatching, and 4) dextran can cause abnormalities in renal tubular cells when given in large doses.

Hetastarch is a starch derivative that is available as a 6% solution in 0.9% sodium chloride. Its colloidal properties are similar to those of albumin, and it has been used as a plasma volume expander in hemorrhagic shock due to trauma. It is not, however, a substitute for blood and has no advantage over the combination of Ringer's lactate plus blood in the fluid volume resuscitation of the trauma patient.

Improving Cardiac Performance

Inotropic Agents If shock remains refractory to adequate volume loading, therapy should be directed at improving cardiac function and vascular tone. An infusion of dopamine should be started. Sometimes it is clinically advantageous to start a low-dose infusion of dopamine while volume replacement is being undertaken. Dopamine in this setting would improve the contractility of the heart and help preserve renal perfusion. It should not be abused, however, since the prime therapy of hypovolemic shock is volume. The patient may also be started on digoxin intravenously. Rarely should another inotropic agent be required in pure hemorrhagic shock. Other agents occasionally used include dobutamine, isoproterenol, epinephrine, and norepinephrine. For details of their administration refer to the section on "Treatment" in Chapter 2.

If shock remains refractory to volume therapy, efforts should be aimed at improving cardiac performance and vascular tone.

How to use bicarbonate therapy

Bicarbonate The patient in extremis from hemorrhagic shock should receive at least one or two ampules (50–100 mEq) of sodium bicarbonate acutely while awaiting the results of arterial blood gas (ABG) analysis. Additional doses can be titrated depending on subsequent ABG measurements. Inotropic agents do not work as well at acidemic pH. It is important, therefore, to correct the metabolic acidemia of severe hemorrhagic shock so that these agents will be effective.

Using calcium chloride

Calcium Calcium is necessary for normal muscle contraction and has a positive inotropic effect on the heart. The level of normal calcium in patients receiving massive amounts of blood transfusions may become low. Any patient receiving 6 units of blood acutely or any patient in cardiac arrest should receive 10 ml of 10% calcium chloride. This may help in the resuscitation of these most critically ill patients.

Case Study

A 16-year-old male is involved in a motorcycle accident. At the scene he is comatose with a blood pressure of 60 mm Hg. A peripheral IV of Ringer's lactate is started, the MAST suit is applied and inflated, and the patient is transported to the emergency room. Upon arrival the patient is noted to have a blood pressure (BP) of 80 mm Hg, pulse 140, agonal respirations, cyanosis, and contusions about the head and left chest. Bleeding and vomitus are noted in the oropharynx, making intubation impossible. An emergency cricothyroidotomy is performed. The patient is hyperventilated on 100% O_2. Another upper extremity large-bore IV is started, a CVP line is inserted via the left subclavian vein, blood work is sent, a Foley catheter is placed, and a gastric tube is placed via the patient's mouth. Two liters of Ringer's lactate is administered over 10–15 minutes. BP is now 95 mm Hg and pulse is 115. Portable skull x-ray, lateral C-spine, chest x-ray, and KUB reveal a left hemopneumothorax and a fractured right femoral neck and acetabulum. A No. 36 chest tube is placed in the left chest and yields 750 ml of blood immediately with no subsequent drainage. The patient is seen in consultation by a general surgeon, a neurosurgeon, and an orthopedic surgeon. The hematocrit returns at 30, and the urinalysis is negative for occult blood. An emergency brain CT scan reveals a left acute subdural hematoma. Concurrently the patient receives 2 units of blood. The patient is next transported to the operating room with the MAST suit still inflated. A simultaneous craniotomy and exploratory laparotomy are performed. A subdural hematoma is evacuated and a massively disrupted spleen is removed. The right leg is subsequently placed in traction.

The above case illustrates the principles of management of the multiple trauma patient in hemorrhagic shock. The important points to note include: 1) priority of airway and breathing and need for cricothyroidotomy; 2) need for multiple IVs and use of Ringer's lactate in initial resuscitation; 3) necessity of the MAST suit in stabilizing hemodynamics and its persistent use to the operating room; 4) shock in multiple trauma is due to bleeding and not to head injury; 5) the expeditious use of consulting services.

One further point needs emphasis. Peritoneal lavage was not performed in this patient. The MAST suit was required for stabilization, and thus removal of the abdominal portion of the suit to perform lavage in the emergency room setting may have jeopardized the patient's hemodynamic profile. Intraabdominal hemorrhage was presumed due to the patient's clinical course. Most surgeons would explore this patient without lavage; however, some, as a compromise, would consider lavage in the operating room to confirm their clinical impression.

Case Study

A 25-year-old man sustains a gunshot wound to the right chest and is brought to the emergency room by private car. The patient is agitated, BP is 75 mm Hg, pulse 140, and respiratory rate 30. A single bullet wound is noted anteriorly at the sixth intercostal space, there are decreased breath sounds over the right chest, and the upper abdomen is tender. Oxygen 100% is administered by mask, two large-bore IVs are inserted in the upper extremities, a No. 36

chest tube is inserted in the right chest, and blood work is sent. About 500 ml of blood returns from the chest tube acutely without further loss. The patient receives 2 liters of Ringer's lactate in about 10 minutes. BP is still 85 and pulse is 130. The MAST suit is applied and inflated and the BP increases to 95. A Foley catheter is placed, as is a nasogastric tube. No hematuria is noted. The patient is seen by a general surgeon and brought to the operating room for laparotomy. Exploration reveals about 1500 ml of intraperitoneal blood, a large wound of the right hepatic lobe, and a small hole in the diaphragm. The bullet is in the right flank, having missed the kidney and the vena cava. Hemostasis is obtained, the liver wound is debrided and drained, and the diaphragm is repaired. Intraoperatively the patient receives 5 units of blood.

The above case illustrates the principles of management of penetrating thoracoabdominal trauma in hemorrhagic shock. Points to note include: 1) priority of airway and breathing, need for O_2 administration, and indication for chest tube insertion; 2) use of multiple IVs and Ringer's lactate solution; 3) use of the MAST suit in penetrating abdominal injury with shock; and 4) need for prompt surgery without superfluous x-ray studies, which would delay definitive care.

Annotated Bibliography

Baker CC, Oppenheimer L, Stephens B, et al. Epidemiology of trauma deaths. Am J Surg 140: 144–150, 1980.

An excellent recent review of the epidemiology of deaths caused by trauma.

Blaisdell TW, Trunkey DD (eds). Trauma Management: Vol. 1, Abdominal Trauma. Thieme-Stratton, New York, 1982.

An exciting, comprehensive survey on the diagnosis and treatment of blunt and penetrating abdominal trauma.

Carey LC, Lowery BD, Cloutier CT. Hemorrhagic shock. Curr Probl Surg, pp 3–48, January 1971.

A review of the treatment of hemorrhagic shock using case studies from the Vietnam experience.

Kaplan BC, Civetta JM, Nagel EL, et al. The military anti-shock trouser in civilian pre-hospital emergency care. J Trauma 13:843–848, 1973.

The first civilian use of the MAST suit.

Levison M, Trunkey PD. Initial assessment and resuscitation. Surg Clin North Am 62:9–16, 1982.

An up-to-date review on the priorities of trauma management.

Meyer AA, Cross RA. Abdominal trauma. Surg Clin North Am 62:105-111, 1982.

A current, succinct review of abdominal injury.

Robinson WA. Fluid therapy in hemorrhagic shock. Crit Care Q 2:11–13, 1980.

An excellent summary of the fluids available in the treatment of hemorrhagic shock.

Shires GT, Canizaro PC. Fluid resuscitation in the severely injured. Surg Clin North Am 53:1341–1366, 1973.

The why and how-to guide to volume therapy in shock.

Zuidema GD, Rutherford RB, Ballinger WF II (eds). The Management of Trauma. W. B. Saunders, Philadelphia, 1979.

The comprehensive textbook on trauma, including a detailed review on the pathophysiology and management of shock.

Additional Bibliography

Archie JP Jr, Mertz WR. Myocardial oxygen delivery after experimental hemorrhagic shock. Ann Surg 187:205–210, 1978.

Baker RJ, Shoemaker WC. Changing concepts in the treatment of hypovolemic shock. Med Clin North Am 51:83–96, 1967.

Baue AE, Tragus ET, Wolfson SK Jr, et al. Hemodynamic and metabolic effects of Ringer's lactate solution in hemorrhagic shock. Ann Surg 116:29–38, 1967.

Burri C, Henkemeyer H, Passelr HH, et al. Evaluation

of acute blood loss by means of simple hemodynamic parameters. Prog Surg 11:109–127, 1973.

Canizaro PC, Prager MD, Shires GT. The infusion of Ringer's lactate solution during shock. Am J Surg 122:494–501, 1971.

Civetta JM, Nussenfeld SR, Rowe TR, et al. Pre-hospital use of the military anti-shock trouser (MAST). J Am Coll Emerg Phys 5:581–587, 1976.

Coran AG, Ballantine TV, Horwitz DL, et al. The effect of crystalloid resuscitation in hemorrhagic shock on acid-base balance: A comparison between normal saline and Ringer's lactate solutions. Surgery 69:874–880, 1971.

Dove DB, Stahl WM, DelGuercio LRM. A five-year review of deaths following urban trauma. J Trauma 20:760–766, 1980.

Gaffney FA, Thal ER, Taylor WF, et al. Hemodynamic effects of medical anti-shock trousers (MAST garment). J Trauma 21:931–937, 1981.

Hoffman JR. External counterpressure and the MAST suit: Current and future roles. Am Emerg Med 9:419–421, 1980.

Lewis FR. Thoracic trauma. Surg Clin North Am 62:97–104, 1982.

Lucas CE. Resuscitation of the injured patient: The three phases of treatment. Surg Clin North Am 57:3–15, 1977.

Moss GS. An argument in favor of electrolyte solution for early resuscitation. Surg Clin North Am 52:3–17, 1972.

Nees JE, Hauser CJ, Shippy C, et al. Comparison of cardiorespiratory effects of crystalline hemoglobin, whole blood, albumin, and Ringer's lactate in the resuscitation of hemorrhagic shock in dogs. Surgery 83:639–647, 1978.

Niinikoski J. Tissue oxygenation in hypovolemic shock. Ann Clin Res 9:151–156, 1977.

Oestern HJ, Trentz O, Hempelmann G, et al. Cardiorespiratory and metabolic patterns in multiple trauma patients. Resuscitation 7:169–184, 1979.

Shires GT. Pathophysiology and fluid replacement in hypovolemic shock. Ann Clin Res 9:144–150, 1977.

Trunkey DD. Overview of trauma. Surg Clin North Am 62:3–7, 1982.

Williams LF Jr. Hemorrhagic shock as a source of unconsciousness. Surg Clin North Am 48:263–272, 1968.

Zollman W, Culpepper RD, Turner MD, et al. Hemorrhagic shock in dogs. Am J Surg 131:298–305, 1976.

Zweifach BW, Fronek A. The interplay of central and peripheral factors in irreversible hemorrhagic shock. Prog Cardiovasc Dis 18:147–180, 1975.

Cardiogenic Shock 4

Overview

Cardiogenic shock is a common clinical problem. The most common cause in the United States is acute myocardial infarction (AMI). AMI may be complicated by ventricular failure. It is important to classify the patient with AMI hemodynamically in regard to the presence or absence of pulmonary congestion (PCWP > 18 mm Hg) and peripheral hypoperfusion (cardiac index < 2.2 liters/min/m²). This classification has both prognostic and therapeutic implications. In general, treating pump failure complicating AMI involves: 1) treating and preventing arrhythmias, 2) reestablishing normovolemia whether with volume loading or unloading, and 3) improving cardiac performance.

▇ Definition

Cardiogenic shock can be defined as that clinical shock syndrome which results from the heart failing to pump blood effectively. The heart fails to produce a cardiac output adequate for survival. This results in the clinical signs of pulmonary congestion, hypoperfusion, and circulatory insufficiency. The most common cause is myocardial ischemia and infarction due to coronary artery disease. The magnitude of this problem is great. In the United States coronary artery disease causes about 675,000 deaths per year. An additional 1.3 million people per year sustain nonfatal myocardial infarction. If one adds to this the number of people who develop cardiogenic shock secondary to congestive heart failure, hemorrhage, or sepsis, the total extent of the problem becomes even more evident.

It is important, therefore, for all physicians to

Coronary artery disease causes 675,000 deaths per year.

111

understand cardiogenic shock. Since acute myocardial infarction (AMI) is the most common cause, the emphasis in this chapter will be on cardiogenic shock complicating AMI.

■ Etiology

There are two basic causes of cardiogenic shock: primary causes and secondary causes.

Primary causes involve pump failure.

Primary causes result from defects in the heart's ability to function as a mechanical pump. As a group they are the most common causes of cardiogenic shock. They include: 1) AMI, 2) cardiac dysrhythmias, 3) congestive heart failure, 4) carditis and cardiomyopathies, and 5) congenital heart disease.

Secondary causes involve obstruction to blood flow.

Secondary causes result from mechanical obstruction to blood flow. They include: 1) pulmonary embolism, 2) pericardial tamponade, 3) vena caval syndromes, 4) tension pneumothorax, 5) intracardiac tumors and thrombi, and 6) dissecting aortic aneurysm.

Cardiogenic shock may also complicate other shock syndromes. If hemorrhagic or septic shock is severe and prolonged, then myocardial ischemia and subsequent infarction may result in the cardiogenic shock syndrome.

Cardiogenic shock complicates 10–15% of all patients hospitalized with AMI.

Cardiogenic shock has a 60–90% mortaility rate.

Cardiogenic shock develops in about 10–15% of all patients hospitalized with AMI. About 50% of patients who die from AMI do so prior to reaching the hospital. The mortality rate of cardiogenic shock in hospitalized patients is between 60 and 90% despite very aggressive therapy. Even among survivors the long-term prognosis is poor, with about 60% dying within 9 months of discharge.

The above statistics are admittedly grim. However, it should be evident that, if the prognosis of heart disease is to be improved, physicians should aggressively monitor, diagnose, and treat lesser forms of circulatory insufficiency (heart failure, hypoperfusion, pulmonary congestion) and cardiac dysrhythmias complicating AMI. An aggressive attitude is the only way that subtle hemodynamic changes can be treated promptly so as to avert the bona fide cardiogenic shock syndrome.

Diagnosis

The antecedent history is important. The patient may relate a history of previous myocardial infarction, angina, hypertension, congestive heart failure, and cardiac arrhythmias. Most patients with AMI will complain of substernal chest pain. This pain may radiate to the neck, jaw, arms, back, and epigastrium. For unknown reasons about 30% of patients with a nonfatal AMI will not have pain. Painless infarction is more common in diabetics, in hypertensives, among blacks, and in chronic atrial fibrillation.

Most patients with AMI have chest pain.

The signs and symptoms of cardiogenic shock are related to the two major hemodynamic alterations that must exist in order for the syndrome to develop. These are: 1) an elevated left ventricular filling pressure as measured clinically by the pulmonary capillary wedge pressure (PCWP) and 2) a decreased cardiac output and cardiac index. These two abnormalities in cardiac hemodynamics are identified clinically as pulmonary congestion and peripheral hypoperfusion.

The hemodynamic alterations and their clinical correlates in cardiogenic shock

Pulmonary congestion is manifested by dyspnea, rales, and cyanosis. An S3 gallop may be heard, indicating an increased left ventricular volume. The jugular veins may be distended and the liver may be enlarged, indicating an elevated right ventricular and right atrial pressure. The chest x-ray will show progressive deterioration as pulmonary congestion worsens. Arterial blood gas analysis will confirm progressive hypoxemia. Peripheral hypoperfusion is manifested by hypotension, oliguria (decreased renal perfusion), obtundation (decreased cerebral perfusion), and cyanosis or pallor (decreased cutaneous perfusion). The pulse may be weak and the carotid upstroke diminished. There may be diaphoresis.

The Swan-Ganz balloon flotation catheter has greatly sophisticated the assessment of heart failure. By using this catheter one can perform objective hemodynamic measurements of pulmonary congestion (via the PCWP) and peripheral hypoperfusion (via the cardiac output and cardiac index).

Use the Swan-Ganz catheter to assess pulmonary congestion (via PCWP) and hypoperfusion (via cardiac output, cardiac index).

The magnitude of pulmonary congestion depends on the PCWP. The normal PCWP is usually less than 12 mm Hg. Pulmonary congestion begins

Pulmonary congestion begins at a PCWP of 18 mm Hg.

when the PCWP reaches 18–20 mm Hg. The normal plasma colloid oncotic pressure is about 25–30 mm Hg. When the PCWP exceeds this level, fluid shifts from the intravascular to the interstitial and eventually to the intra-alveolar space. Thus, pulmonary edema usually occurs when the PCWP exceeds 30 mm Hg.

Peripheral hypoperfusion begins when the cardiac index decreases below 2.2 liters/min/m².

The magnitude of peripheral hypoperfusion depends on the cardiac index. Normal cardiac index is 3.0 ± 0.5 liters/min/m². Peripheral hypoperfusion begins when the cardiac index decreases to 2.2 liters/min/m². Frank cardiogenic shock results when the cardiac index is less than 1.8 liters/min/m².

From the above it is clear that the initial clinical manifestations of heart failure occur at specific hemodynamic levels of cardiac preload (PCWP) and cardiac index. Pulmonary congestion begins at a PCWP of 18 mm Hg, and peripheral hypoperfusion begins at a cardiac index of 2.2 liters/min/m². These two hemodynamic measurements, therefore, define when clinical heart failure may develop.

Cardiac function is variable in AMI.

In AMI there is much individual patient-to-patient variation in cardiac function. Some patients with AMI will present with a normal PCWP and a normal cardiac index. Other patients may present with varying degrees of pulmonary congestion and peripheral hypoperfusion. Some patients will present in cardiogenic shock. These different hemodynamic subsets following AMI will be discussed fully in the next section, "Pathophysiology."

About 25% of patients post-AMI have a cardiac index less than 2.2 liters/min/m² despite absence of clinical signs of hypoperfusion.

About 15% of patients post-AMI have PCWP above 18 mm Hg despite absence of clinical signs of pulmonary congestion.

Cardiogenic shock is usually an easily recognizable syndrome. It is with lesser degrees of heart failure that clinical assessment alone of the hemodynamic profile may be inaccurate. It has been estimated that about 25% of patients who are deemed clinically to have normal perfusion post-AMI actually have cardiac indices less than 2.2 liters/min/m². Moreover, in about 15% of patients post-AMI the physician clinically fails to diagnose a PCWP elevated above 18 mm Hg. The clinical reliability in diagnosing both early pulmonary congestion and peripheral hypoperfusion after an AMI is only about 80%.

Accurate hemodynamic assessment using a Swan-Ganz catheter is extremely important. This catheter need not be inserted into every patient with AMI. However, one's threshold for doing so should be very low. As stated earlier, it is hoped that, by identifying those patients with hemodynamic evidence for heart failure, the cardiogenic shock syndrome might be preventable for some patients.

There should be a low threshold for inserting a Swan-Ganz catheter.

Further comments about the diagnosis of AMI are warranted. The clinical history and physical examination are obviously important. The EKG, however, is nondiagnostic in at least 20% of cases. ST segment elevation usually resolves in 36–48 hours but on occasion may persist for 1–2 weeks. If the ST segment remains elevated beyond this time period, there is about a 60% chance that a ventricular aneurysm has developed secondary to AMI. Q waves may occur early. Serial EKG analysis is therefore important.

The EKG in AMI

The measurement of serum creatinine phosphokinase (CPK) isoenzyme (MB fraction) is an extremely accurate way to assess the occurrence of AMI. The MB fraction comes mainly from cardiac muscle. Normal CPK-MB is less than 2–4%. A CPK-MB fraction greater than 4% is usually indicative of AMI. Peak levels of CPK-MB are usually noted at about 20 hours postinfarction, and most of the enzyme disappears from serum at about 2 days. It is recommended, therefore, that this enzyme be measured on admission to the hospital and every 8–12 hours thereafter for three additional determinations.

The use of CPK isoenzyme

A CPK-MB > 4% is indicative of AMI.

It is no longer necessary to measure serum glutamine oxaloacetate transaminase (SGOT) or lactic dehydrogenase (LDH) levels to diagnose AMI, with one exception. If the patient presents to the hospital 2 days or more postinfarction, the CPK-MB level may be normal. The EKG may likewise be normal. In this instance measuring LDH isoenzymes (LDH_1, LDH_2) might make the diagnosis of AMI. Normally the serum concentration of LDH_2 is greater than LDH_1. In AMI this ratio is reversed and may persist reversed for 6 days.

Occasionally LDH isoenzymes are helpful.

AMI may also be diagnosed using radioisotope scanning. The technetium-99m pyrophosphate scan becomes positive about 12 hours postinfarction and persists for up to 6 days. This scan has a greater than 90% accuracy. The thallium-201 scan becomes posi-

Scanning in the diagnosis of AMI

tive at about 6 hours postinfarction but persists for only about 24 hours. The accuracy of this scan is about 80%.

▰ Pathophysiology

The pathophysiology of cardiogenic shock involves failure of the left ventricle to function adequately as a mechanical pump. There is a marked decrease in the contractile state of the left ventricle. In AMI this decreased contractility is due to actual necrosis of the myocardium from inadequate nutrient myocar-

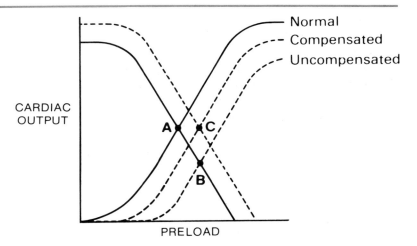

FIGURE 4.1   Cardiogenic shock due to myocardial infarction results from an acute decrease in myocardial contractility and cardiac performance. The ventricular function curve shifts downward and to the right, causing a new equilibrium point (B). The body compensates by: 1) increasing blood volume (via venoconstriction, ADH, aldosterone) and 2) improving cardiac inotropy (via sympathetic nervous system, epinephrine). The systemic function curve shifts upward and to the right, while the ventricular function curve shifts upward and to the left. The compensated equilibrium point (C) represents an improved hemodynamic state over point B. Adapted with permission from Kelman GR Applied Cardiovascular Physiology. Butterworths, Woburn MA, 1977, p 126.

dial blood flow. Necrotic muscle cannot contract. It has been estimated that when cardiogenic shock complicates AMI at least 40% of the left ventricle muscle mass has been infarcted. Obviously this is a major injury. The resultant decrease in left ventricular contractility can be viewed as a rightward shift in the ventricular function curve. In cardiogenic shock this curve may approach the horizontal in that the cardiac output changes little regardless of the preloading conditions placed on the left ventricle.

When cardiogenic shock complicates AMI, at least 40% of the left ventricle has been infarcted.

Apart from frank infarction, ischemia too causes a rapid decrease in the contractility of the left ventricle. It is known that after only 2–3 minutes of cardiac ischemia the rate of myocardial glycolysis is only about 25% of normal. This causes a decrease in myocardial ATP production. Ischemic myocardium will lose its contractility.

Ischemia too causes a decrease in contractility.

In most patients with AMI there is a decrease in cardiac performance. The equilibrium point on the ventricular function curve will accordingly shift from point A to point B (Figure 4.1). Whether or not the infarcted area is compliant or noncompliant will determine also the severity of altered cardiac performance. With a compliant infarct the affected area will take up some of the stroke volume so that cardiac output is decreased even further. This paradoxical bulging of the infarcted zone is called asynergy and can be visualized at cardiac catheterization. If the infarcted zone is noncompliant, then more of the ventricular and diastolic volume can be delivered to the aorta during systole. A noncompliant infarction thus has a mechanical advantage over a compliant infarction.

A noncompliant infarct has a mechanical edge over a compliant infarct.

Various compensatory homeostatic mechanisms are activated during failure. As in hemorrhagic shock, these mechanisms include: 1) hemodynamic adjustments and 2) hormonal adjustments. Hypotension from decreased cardiac output causes activation of the sympathetic nervous system. This system then produces: 1) vasoconstriction, 2) venoconstriction, 3) increased cardiac contractility and heart rate, and 4) redistribution of blood flow to heart and brain. Vasoconstriction increases peripheral resistance and thus blood pressure. Venoconstriction augments cardiac preload. This is important, for up

There are hemodynamic and hormonal adjustments to pump failure.

Twenty percent of patients with AMI are hypovolemic.

to 20% of patients with AMI are initially hypovolemic. This may be due to diaphoresis, vomiting, or diuretic therapy. Augmenting cardiac preload via venoconstriction may serve as a useful mechanism to improve cardiac performance in some patients. Improved contractility and heart rate tend to augment cardiac output. Hormonal adjustments involve secretion of epinephrine, aldosterone, and ADH. Epinephrine serves as an endogenous vasopressor and also increases cardiac contractility and heart rate. Aldosterone and ADH act to conserve water and salt. Preload may thus be increased further.

Compensation can be viewed graphically.

The compensatory mechanisms function in order to improve cardiac output and blood pressure. This may be viewed graphically using the ventricular function curve (Figure 4.1). With pump failure the equilibrium point shifts from point A to point B such that for each level of ventricular preload there is diminished cardiac output. Improved contractility (via sympathetic nervous system, epinephrine) will shift the ventricular function curve to a better hemodynamic position, that is, to the left. Improved preload (via venoconstriction, ADH, aldosterone) will shift the systemic function curve to the right. A new equilibrium, point C, results. In compensated heart failure, therefore, there is some improvement in cardiac performance for each level of preload, although point A is not reached.

The compensatory mechanism may eventually have an adverse effect on the heart.

The above analysis helps one understand the homeostatic mechanisms that come into play to correct pump failure. This analysis is general, however. Indeed, most patients with AMI are not hypovolemic. In addition, in severe pump failure these compensatory mechanisms may eventually have a deleterious effect on cardiac hemodynamics. Increasing the heart rate, contractile state, preload (ventricular size), and blood pressure (afterload) all increase myocardial oxygen demand. This may increase the zone of ischemia or infarction and cause further deterioration in cardiac performance.

Myocardial ischemia and infarction cause structural cardiac damage.

Apart from their effects on contractility, myocardial ischemia and infarction may cause structural damage to the heart and thereby cause cardiogenic shock. Papillary muscle dysfunction may occur secondary to papillary muscle ischemia, infarction, rupture, ventricular asynergy, and ventricular dilatation. Papillary muscle dysfunction causes mitral regurgitation and a holosystolic murmur.

The diagnosis of acute mitral regurgitation complicating AMI can be made using the Swan-Ganz catheter. With the catheter in the wedge position a giant V wave is noted in the PCWP tracing. The giant V wave reflects the marked increase in left atrial pressure during systole because of mitral regurgitation. Mitral regurgitation has a very adverse affect on cardiac performance. For example, it is known that a 40% infarct has the same hemodynamic profile as a 10% infarct that is complicated by moderate mitral regurgitation.

Acute mitral regurgitation and ventricular septal rupture may complicate AMI and may mandate surgery.

A ruptured ventricular septum may occasionally complicate AMI. As in papillary muscle dysfunction with mitral regurgitation, a holosystolic murmur is heard with a perforated ventricular septum. The Swan-Ganz catheter can again be used to diagnose this condition. A step-up in O_2 saturation is noted from the right atrium to the pulmonary artery. It is important to identify these drastic sequelae of AMI, as the definitive treatment is often early surgery.

In AMI there are a variety of possible hemodynamic subsets. It is important to classify each individual patient within one of the hemodynamic subsets so that apropriate therapeutic intervention can be undertaken. The classification system developed by Forrester and associates is most pertinent to this end. These investigators have identified four clinical and hemodynamic subsets (Table 4.1).

In AMI there are four hemodynamic and clinical subsets.

Subset 1 includes those patients with either normal or hyperdynamic hemodynamics. There is no pulmonary congestion or peripheral hypoperfusion. The PCWP is less than 18 mm Hg, and the

TABLE 4.1   Hemodynamic Subsets in Myocardial Infarction

	Pulmonary Congestion (PCWP > 18 mm Hg.)	*Peripheral Hypoperfusion (CI < 2.2 liters/min/m²)*	*Mortality (percentage)*
Subset I	No	No	1%
Subset II	Yes	No	10
Subset III	No	Yes	20
Subset IV (cardiogenic shock)	Yes	Yes	60

Adapted with permission from Forrester JS, Diamond G, Chattergie K., and Swan, H. medical therapy of acute myocardial infarction by application of hemodynamic subsets. N Eng J Med 295:1361, 1976.

About one-third of patients with AMI have normal or hyperdynamic hemodynamics when first seen.

cardiac index is greater than 2.2 liters/min/m². About one-third of AMI patients are in this subset when initially evaluated. Subset II identifies those patients with pulmonary congestion but without peripheral hypoperfusion. The PCWP is greater than 18 mm Hg, and the cardiac index is greater than 2.2 liters/min/m². Subset III consists of those patients without pulmonary congestion but with peripheral hypoperfusion. The PCWP is less than 18 mm Hg, and the cardiac index is less than 2.2 liters/min/m². Subset IV identifies those patients with both pulmonary congestion and peripheral hypoperfusion. The PCWP is greater than 18 mm Hg, and the cardiac index is less than 2.2 liters/min/m². Cardiogenic shock is a

Initial subset classification is prognostic.

part of subset IV. The approximate mortality rates for each subset are as follows: subset I, 1%, subset II, 10%; subset III, 20%; and subset IV, 60%. The application of this hemodynamic subset classification will become evident in the next section, "Treatment."

Cardiac rhythm disturbances occur in 90% of patients with AMI.

About 90% of patients with AMI develop some disturbance in cardiac rhythm. Much of the decrease in mortality from AMI in recent years is a direct result of the aggressive monitoring, diagnosis, and treatment of cardiac arrhythmias. Several points should be emphasized. Over 90% of patients who die within 1 hour of AMI are found to have ventricular fibrillation. Over 80% of patients with AMI when first seen will have either tachycardia (via sympathetic stimulation) or bradycardia (via parasympathetic stimulation). Bradycardia is more common with inferior infarction. It may cause hypotension. Untreated bradycardia hypotension complicating AMI causes a 75% prehospital mortality. Heart block too is more common with inferior infarction. Complete heart block complicating AMI

Seventy-five percent of AMI patients develop premature ventricular contractions.

has a 50% mortaility. About 75% of AMI patients develop premature ventricular contractions. Lethal arrhythmias like ventricular fibrillation may occur without warning. Indeed, one study has found no warning dysrhythmias in 40% of cases of ventricular fibrillation. It is clear from the above that all patients with AMI should be monitored by continuous EKG. There is good evidence to support the use of prophylactic antiarrhythmic drugs in AMI.

The treatment of cardiac ischemia, AMI, and cardiogenic shock should include increasing myocardial O_2 supply and decreasing myocardial O_2 demands. By so doing, the ischemia tone may be reversed and the size of actual infarction may be contained. The myocardial O_2 supply is equal to the product of coronary blood flow times the amount of O_2 extracted per milliliter of blood. The myocardium extracts 65–70% of the O_2 delivered to it at rest. This cannot be improved upon. Thus, in order to effectively increase O_2 supply to the myocardium the coronary blood flow must be increased. This is physiologically difficult in the presence of coronary artery disease.

The determinants of myocardial O_2 supply

Coronary blood flow is normally regulated by changes in coronary vascular resistance. In cardiogenic shock and AMI, however, the amount of coronary blood flow is relatively fixed. There are several reasons for this. The coronary arteries are diseased, stenotic, obstructed, and rigid. Associated tachycardia will limit coronary flow, since more of the cardiac cycle is spent in systole whereas most (70%) of coronary flow occurs in diastole. Finally, with heart failure the ventricular wall tension increases. This too will inhibit coronary blood flow.

There are four hemodynamic variables that increase myocardial O_2 demands. They are: 1) arterial pressure (afterload), 2) heart size (preload), 3) contractility, and 4) heart rate. The therapy of cardiogenic shock includes decreasing some of these O_2 demands while others are increased. In cardiogenic shock, therapy is aimed at increasing the blood pressure, improving the contractile state of the myocardium, establishing normal heart rate, and lowering an elevated filling pressure (preload, PCWP). By improving the overall hemodynamic profile it is hoped that the myocardial O_2 demands are not greatly increased. If the myocardial O_2 demands persistently exceed O_2 supply, then there may occur extension of the ischemic zone and infarct size.

The hemodynamic variables that increase myocardial O_2 demands

▬ Treatment

Treating cardiogenic shock or pump failure complicating AMI involves three primary avenues of the therapy: 1) preventing ventricular arrhythmias and treating any existing arrhythmias, 2) reestablishing

The goals of therapy in cardiogenic shock include:
1) Prevent arrhythmias: prophylactic lidocaine
2) Reestablish normovolemia
   a) Volume loading: crystalloid
   b) Volume unloading: diuretics
                          nitroprusside
                          nitroglycerin
                          morphine
                          phlebotomy
3) Improve cardiovascular performance
   a) Inotropic agents
   b) Sodium bicarbonate
   c) Calcium chloride
   d) MAST suit
   e) Vasopressor agents
   f) Intra-aortic balloon pump
   g) Cardiac surgery

normovolemia, and 3) improving cardiac performance. Attention must be directed at correcting all three parameters if resuscitative efforts are to be successful.

Assure adequate respiratory status.

As in any resuscitative effort, control of the airway and assuring adequate ventilation are the first objectives. Once attained, attention can then be directed at the circulation. These critically ill patients should be monitored using a Swan-Ganz catheter, an arterial pressure cannula, a Foley catheter, and a continuous EKG monitor. Only by identifying specific hemodynamic profiles can appropriate therapy be instituted. These monitoring devices are necessary in identifying specific hemodynamic profiles.

Reestablishing normovolemia may involve either volume loading in the hypovolemic patient or volume unloading in the hypervolemic patient. Volume unloading, so that the PCWP decreases to less than 18 mm Hg, is necessary to correct pulmonary congestion. Improving cardiac performance involves using those drugs that increase cardiac output and peripheral perfusion. This may include some combination of inotropic agent, vasopressor, or vasodilator therapy.

As stated previously, about 90% of patients with AMI develop cardiac arrhythmias of one kind or another. It is recommended, therefore, that all patients with AMI receive antiarrhythmic prophylaxis using lidocaine. Some cardiologists recommend that lidocaine be administered prophylactically in the pre-hospital phase of illness by paramedical ambulance personnel. The drug can achieve good plasma levels using a single intramuscular injection (deltoid muscle) of 4 mg/kg lidocaine. There are conflicting reports, however, about the benefits of this treatment.

Prophylactic antiar-rhythmic therapy is indicated in AMI.

It has been shown, on the other hand, that the prophylactic intravenous use of lidocaine in the hospital after AMI lessens the risk of developing ventricular fibrillation. All patients with AMI should receive lidocaine prophylactically for 48–72 hours. Various regimens for administering the drug have been proposed. The half-life of a bolus injection is only 9 minutes. It is necessary to start a continuous infusion of lidocaine after bolus therapy. One straightforward method of administration involves an initial bolus dose of 1 mg/kg. This is followed immediately by a 4-mg/min continuous infusion. It has been shown that if a 2-mg/min continuous infusion is selected following a 1-mg/kg bolus dose, the plasma levels become subtherapeutic in 100% of patients at 15 minutes. It is important, therefore, to use the higher 4-mg/min continuous infusion. Lidocaine therapy should continue for 48 hours, and then the patient is weaned off the drug.

Lidocaine should be given for 48–72 hours post-AMI.

The dose of lidocaine

Bradycardia-hypotension after AMI should be vigorously treated with atropine. Atropine can be used to treat sinus bradycardia or initially in the treatment of heart block. It is administered as 0.5 mg IV every 3–5 minutes for a total dose of 2 mg. If bradycardia persists, a drip infusion of isoproterenol (1 mg/500 ml) may be tried. Isoproterenol should not be used for long time periods because it greatly increases the myocardial O_2 demand. If bradycardia-hypotension remains refractory to atropine and isoproterenol, then a temporary transvenous cardiac pacemaker should be inserted. This can be accomplished via the subclavian, internal jugular, or femoral vein routes. These catheters are now equipped with inflatable balloons at their distal ends, which allow them to flow into the right ventricle. This has simplified the ease of their insertion, which can on occasion be accomplished at the bedside without fluoroscopy.

The treatment of bradycardia-hypotension

The treatment of premature ventricular contractions

About 75% of patients with AMI develop premature ventricular contractions. These are always significant, but certain patterns have greater potential for developing ventricular tachycardia or fibrillation. These include closely coupled premature ventricular contractions, multifocal premature ventricular contractions, and R-on-T phenomena. Lidocaine is the drug of choice in the therapy of premature ventricular contractions. A bolus dose of 1 mg/kg is followed by a continuous infusion of 4 mg/min. If the arrhythmia persists, procainamide should be used. It is administered as 100-mg aliquots IV every 5 minutes until either the arrhythmia ceases or a total dose of 1 g has been given. Once the arrhythmia is suppressed, a continuous infusion of 1–4 mg/min should be started. When using bolus doses of procainamide it is important to monitor closely the EKG and blood pressure.

If premature ventricular contractions persist despite lidocaine and procainamide—an uncommon occurrence—then other drugs should be tried. These agents include bretylium, verapamil, diphenylhydantoin, and propranolol. Ventricular tachycardia should be treated immediately with a precordial thump, intravenous lidocaine, and, if necessary, precordial shock using 400 watt-seconds in the adult. Ventricular fibrillation should be treated immediately with a precordial shock followed by an infusion of lidocaine.

Most supraventricular tachyarrhythmias complicating AMI are best treated with intravenous digoxin. On occasion other drugs like quinidine, verapamil, procainamide, or propranolol are required. If these tachyarrhythmias cause hypotension or cardiogenic shock, immediate precordial shock is indicated.

Upon initial hemodynamic investigation about 20% of patients with AMI are hypovolemic. If these patients have peripheral hypoperfusion (hypotension, decreased cardiac output, oliguria, cardiogenic shock), then much can be gained by fluid volume therapy. The hemodynamic profile will improve with volume loading. This is due to the influence of preload on stroke volume and cardiac output. Volume loading shifts the systemic function curve to the right

Volume therapy in AMI

so that a new, hemodynamically improved equilibrium point is reached (Figure 4.1).

Increments of fluid volume are administered while the PCWP, blood pressure, and urine output are being monitored. Cardiac output may also be monitored. The PCWP is used as an accurate guide to fluid therapy and volume loading of the left ventricle. Fluid is administered as bolus therapy (100–250 ml) every 10–15 minutes while the above parameters are being monitored. The end point is normovolemia (PCWP 15–18 mm Hg). If peripheral hypoperfusion persists despite reestablishment of normovolemia, then therapy should be directed at the heart and peripheral vessels. Various fluids can be used as volume loading agents. Most commonly used fluids include normal saline, Ringer's lactate, albumin, and FFP. In the anemic patient blood transfusions can be used. The use of dextran can no longer be recommended for this purpose.

The hemodynamic subsets identified in AMI by Forrester and associates help one's understanding of an effective, rational treatment program. About one-third of all patients with AMI have either a normal or a hyperdynamic hemodynamic profile (subset I). There is no pulmonary congestion (PCWP < 18 mm Hg) and no peripheral hypoperfusion (cardiac index [CI] > 2.2 liters/min/m^2). In general, therapy of patients in this subset is expectant only.

About 50% of patients with AMI are in heart failure when first evaluated. The signs of heart failure include pulmonary congestion and peripheral hypoperfusion. There may be pulmonary congestion (PCWP > 18 mm Hg) without peripheral hypoperfusion (CI > 2.2 liters/min/m^2; subset II), peripheral hypoperfusion (CI < 2.2 liters/min/m^2) without pulmonary congestion (PCWP < 18 mm Hg; subset III), and both pulmonary congestion (PCWP > 18 mm Hg) and peripheral hypoperfusion (CI < 2.2 liters/min/m^2; subset IV). Cardiogenic shock is part of subset IV. The presence of peripheral hypoperfusion markedly increases the mortality rate.

For those patients with pulmonary congestion without peripheral hypoperfusion (subset II), therapy is aimed at lowering the PCWP to the 15- to 18-mm Hg range. This is mainly accomplished using

Identify hemodynamic subsets.

About one-third of patients are in subset I and require expectant treatment only.

About one-half of patients are in heart failure when first evaluated after AMI.

Cardiogenic shock is part of subset IV.

Treatment of those with pulmonary congestion but no peripheral hypoperfusion

Diuretics to treat pulmonary congestion

diuretic therapy. An intravenous dose of furosemide (0.5–1.0 mg/kg) can cause a 25% decrease in the PCWP in 30 minutes. There is little change in cardiac output. Decreasing the preload in this fashion decreases the left ventricular size and thus the myocardial O_2 demand. There is a lag phase, however, between this hemodynamic improvement and improvement in the clinical picture. It may take between 12 and 48 hours to resolve pulmonary rales and x-ray evidence of pulmonary congestion despite establishment of normovolemia. Overzealous use of diuretic agents is avoidable by monitoring the PCWP.

The use of digoxin in AMI

Inotropic agents and vasodilating agents also decrease ventricular preload and pulmonary congestion. There is controversy in the literature concerning the use of digoxin in AMI patients. Digoxin has a positive inotropic effect on the remaining normal and ischemic myocardium in AMI. This increased myocardial contractility may increase the myocardial O_2 demand. On the other hand, preload may be subsequently reduced, and this would tend to decrease the myocardial O_2 demand. If pulmonary congestion remains refractory to diuretic therapy or a supraventricular tachycardia complicates AMI, it seems wise to use digoxin. Furthermore, there is some evidence to suggest that the dose of digoxin necessary to produce a toxic arrhythmia may be decreased in AMI. Therefore, the digitalizing dose should probably be reduced by one-third in AMI.

Inotropic therapy with dopamine may be needed.

Dopamine may also be used to decrease ventricular preload. It does so by: 1) improving contractility and 2) causing renal vasodilation and subsequent diuresis. To maximize these beneficial effects the dose of dopamine should be kept low (0.5–10 μg/kg/min). Dobutamine is a newer inotropic agent that can improve myocardial contractility (and lower PCWP) and is not known to increase infarct size in AMI. The usual starting dose is 2.5–5.0 μg/kg/min.

The use of vasodilators in AMI

Vasodilating agents are also beneficial in treating pulmonary congestion complicating AMI. They do so by either lowering afterload (vasodilators) or lowering preload (venodilators) or both. Decreasing afterload increases stroke volume and cardiac output. Venodilation will decrease venous return and cardiac preload. The PCWP will subsequently decrease. Both of these effects will decrease the myocardial O_2 demand. This application is particularly useful in the patient with pulmonary congestion and hypertension after AMI. Sodium nitroprusside is the most widely used agent for this purpose. It relaxes all vascular smooth muscle and causes both vasodilation and venodilation. Cardiac output improves and PCWP decreases. Nitroprusside infusion should start at 8–16 µg/min. Most patients eventually require 50–150 µg/min as a continuous drip. Intravenous nitroglycerin can also be used. It is mainly a venodilator. Dosages should start at 10 µg/min continuous infusion. Various oral preparations may also be used. Nitroglycerin may be given sublingually (doses of 0.3–0.4 mg). Isosorbide dinitrate also acts like nitroglycerin. It may be given as 2.5–20 mg sublingually every 1–2 hours or 20–80 mg orally every 4 hours. Nitroglycerin may be used as a topical paste with a dose of 1–4 inches applied to the chest every 4 hours. Other agents that may be used orally to produce vasodilation are hydralazine, minoxidil, and prazosin.

The use of nitroprusside

The use of nitroglycerin

For those patients with peripheral hypoperfusion and no pulmonary congestion (subset III), initial therapy involves volume loading so as to maximize ventricular preload. If this is unsuccessful, then attention should be directed at improving contractility and decreasing afterload. Both of these modalities improve stroke volume and, therefore, cardiac output. Contractility may be improved by using digoxin, dopamine, or dobutamine. Afterload reduction is accomplished by using an infusion of sodium nitroprusside, although other agents are occasionally selected.

Treatment of those with peripheral hypoperfusion but no pulmonary congestion

Patients with both pulmonary congestion and peripheral hypoperfusion (subset IV) accompanying AMI have a greater than 50% mortality rate. Treatment must be expedient in this group of patients if survival rates are to improve. Pulmonary congestion is treated by intravenous diuretics (decreasing blood volume, preload) like furosemide. Vasodilator therapy is also indicated. Sodium nitropursside has the dual benefit of decreasing pulmonary congestion by decreasing preload (via venodilation) and by improving cardiac output (by decreasing afterload via

Combining dopamine and nitroprusside may be beneficial for this group of patients.

vasodilation). Inotropic agents like dopamine should also be used to improve contractility and cardiac output. The combination of dopamine and nitroprusside is very beneficial for this group of patients. Occasionally a vasopressor, like norepinephrine, must be used if the patient remains hypotensive despite the foregoing therapy.

The use of the IABP in refractory cardiogenic shock

If cardiogenic shock remains refractory to medical therapy, the insertion of an intra-aortic balloon pump (IABP) may be life-saving. The IABP is inserted via a femoral artery into the descending thoracic aorta. The volume of the balloon varies from 30 to 50 ml. The balloon inflates during diastole and deflates prior to systole. Aortic diastolic pressure is thereby increased (as is coronary artery perfusion), and aortic systolic pressure is decreased (thus lowering afterload). Coronary perfusion and cardiac output are improved by this device. The IABP will help sustain the patient in shock after AMI and while the patient is awaiting definitive cardiac surgery, whether emergent coronary revascularization, repair of septal rupture, or valve replacement.

Case Study

A 68-year-old man undergoes a subtotal gastrectomy for stomach cancer. Intraoperatively he receives 3 units of blood and 3.5 liters of Ringer's lactate. In the recovery room he becomes acutely hypotensive with BP 70 mm Hg, tachycardic with pulse rate 120, and tachypneic with respiratory rate 40. He is immediately reintubated and placed on 100% FIO_2. The CVP measures 10 cm H_2O. Ringer's lactate is given via two wide-open IVs. An ABG and hematocrit are sent to the lab. He receives 500 ml fluid in 5 minutes. The BP rises to 85 mm Hg. A stat EKG shows an ischemic pattern across the precordial leads consistent with an AMI. A stat chest x-ray shows mild cardiomegaly, but the film is taken supine. After 30 minutes the patient has received a total of 1500 ml fluid. The BP is still only 90 mm Hg and the CVP is now 20 cm H_2O. Dopamine infusion is started at 10 mg/kg/min. The BP increases to 100 mm Hg over 5 minutes. The hematocrit returns at 30. A unit of blood is begun. A Swan-Ganz catheter is next inserted and reveals a PCWP of 10 mm Hg. An additional unit of blood is transfused. The BP is now 115 mm Hg and pulse rate 110. The PCWP increases to 15 mm Hg. The patient is transferred to the surgical intensive care unit for further treatment. CPK-MB fraction is ultimately positive for an AMI.

This case represents a common clinical problem, namely, the hypotensive geriatric patient after a major surgical procedure. The common causes of hypotension in this setting include: 1) hypovolemia or hemorrhage, 2) myocardial infarction, 3) pulmonary embolism, and 4) respiratory insufficiency. Several points are warranted: 1) attention is appropriately directed at reestablishing an airway and administering oxygen; 2) hypovolemia is initially assumed and confirmed by the CVP reading; 3) initial fluid resuscitation involves crystalloid therapy with Ringer's lactate; 4) an EKG confirms a probable infarction; 5) dopamine is started once correction of the volume deficit fails to yield hemodynamic stability; 6) Swan-Ganz monitoring reveals that the patient can tolerate additional volume increments to augment ventricular preload.

Annotated Bibliography

Forrester JS, Swan HJC. Acute myocardial infarction: A physiologic basis of therapy. Crit Care Med 2:283–292, 1974.
The basis for treating acute myocardial infarction using physiologic parameters.

Forrester JS, Diamond G, Chatterjee K, Swan H. Medical therapy of acute myocardial infarction by application of hemodynamic subsets. N Engl J Med 295:1356–1362, 1404–1413, 1976.
A classic paper describing in detail the hemodynamic subsets of acute myocardial infarction using the Swan-Ganz catheter: a rational basis for therapy.

Gunnar RM, Loeb HS, Rahimtoola SH (ed). Shock in Myocardial Infarction. Grune & Stratton, New York, 1974.
A detailed text on the hemodynamic alterations in myocardial infarction and its treatment.

Kones RJ. Cardiogenic Shock: Mechanisms and Management. Futura, Mount Kisco NY, 1974.
A comprehensive textbook on cardiogenic shock.

Lester RM, Wagner GS. Acute myocardial infarction. Med Clin North Am 63:3–24, 1979.
A concise review article on acute myocardial infarction.

Additional Bibliography

Arnsdorf MR. Electrophysiologic properties of antidysrhythmic drugs as a rational basis for therapy. Med Clin North Am 60:213–231, 1976.

Chatterjee K. Pump failure in acute myocardial infarction: Fluid and drug therapy. Ann Clin Res 9:124–133, 1977.

Hackel DB, Ratliff NB, Mikat E. The heart in shock. Circ Res 35:805–811, 1974.

Heikkila J. Pump failure and hemodynamic subsets in acute myocardial infarction. Ann Clin Res 9:112–123, 1977.

Hinshaw LB, Archer LT, Black MR, et al. Myocardial function in shock. Am J Physiol 226:357–366, 1974.

Killip T. Arrhythmias in myocardial infarction. Med Clin North Am 60:233–244, 1975.

Kones RJ. Cardiogenic shock. Angiology 25:317–333, 1974.

Kuhn LA. Shock in myocardial infarction—Medical treatment. Am J Cardiol 26:578–587, 1970.

Kuhn LA. Management of shock following acute myocardial infarction. Am Heart J 95:529–534, 789–795, 1978.

Loeb HS, Rahimtoola SH, Gunnar RM. The failing myocardium. Med Clin North Am 57:167–185, 1973.

Luz PL, Weil MH, Shubin H. Current concepts on mechanisms and treatment of cardiogenic shock. Am Heart J 92:103–113, 1976.

Massie BM, Chatterjee K. Vasodilator therapy of pump failure complicating acute myocardial infarction. Med Clin North Am 63:25–51, 1979.

McHugh TJ, Forrester JS, Adler L, et al. Pulmonary vascular congestion in acute myocardial infarction: Hemodynamic and radiologic correlations. Ann Intern Med 76:29–33, 1972.

Norris RM, Mercer CJ. Significance of idioventricular rhythms in acute myocardial infarction. Prog Cardiovasc Dis 16:455–468, 1974.

Park GD. Cardiogenic shock. Crit Care Q 2:43–54, 1980.

Rahimtoola SH, Gunnar RM. Digitalis in acute myocardial infarction: Help or hazard? Ann Intern Med 82:234–240, 1975.

Resnekov L. Circulatory support and early cardiac surgery in the management of cardiogenic shock complicating myocardial infarction. Ann Clin Res 9:134–143, 1977.

Ylikahri RH. Cardiac metabolism in myocardial ischemia. Ann Clin Res 9:102–111, 1977.

Septic Shock 5

Overview

Sepsis is a common clinical problem. Septic shock is the clinical shock syndrome that may complicate sepsis. Gram-negative bacteria are the most common cause of sepsis and septic shock. Septic shock caused by Gram-negative bacteria carries a greater than 50% mortality risk despite all known medical and surgical therapy. Endotoxin probably plays a dominant role in the pathogenesis of Gram-negative septic shock. The treatment of sepsis and septic shock involves: 1) eradicating the infection by antimicrobial agents and/or surgery as needed, 2) reestablishing normovolemia, 3) improving cardiovascular performance, and 4) use of corticosteroids.

▓ Definition

The association of circulatory insufficiency with infection was first made by Laennec in 1831. It is only during the past 30 years, however, that the entity of Gram-negative bacteremia and septic shock has become a major health problem. In the United States nowadays septic shock is a more common cause of death than motor vehicle accidents. The reasons for this are several and include: 1) the widespread use of broad-spectrum antibiotics, 2) the emergence of resistant bacterial strains, and 3) the modern ability to treat and sustain those with lowered host resistance, critical illness, and infection.

Several terms need specific definition. Bacteremia is the invasion of the bloodstream by bacterial pathogens. Sepsis and septicemia are broader terms that imply not only bloodstream invasion but also the subsequent development of clinical symptoms, such as fever or chills. Sepsis may result from blood infection by bacteria, fungi, parasites, rickettsia, or

Defining bacteremia, sepsis, septicemia, septic shock, and endotoxic shock

135

viruses. Septic shock is the clinical shock syndrome that may occur during sepsis. Once the pathogen is identified, one can be specific when describing the clinical septic state. For example, there may occur Gram-negative bacterial sepsis, Gram-negative bacterial septic shock, *Candida* sepsis, etc. The term endotoxic shock should be reserved properly for that shock syndrome that results from the experimental injection of bacterial endotoxin.

This chapter will discuss the etiology, diagnosis, pathophysiology, and treatment of septic shock. Emphasis will be placed on septic shock caused by Gram-negative bacteria.

▆▆▆ Etiology

The determinants of sepsis include the specific pathogen, the environment, and the host's defense mechanisms.

As in any infection there are three major determinants of bacterial sepsis: the bacterial pathogen, the environment (or site of infection), and the host's defense mechanisms. Alterations in the normal homeostatic balance among these factors may cause sepsis. For example, it is known that, once hospitalized, a patient's normal, endogenous flora, particularly of the skin and oronasopharynx, is replaced over a few days by exogenous hospital flora. These organisms are more pathogenic and more resistant to antibiotics than are the endogenous flora. They are also predominantly Gram-negative. Most nosocomial, or hospital-acquired pneumonias, therefore, are Gram-negative. This is in contrast with community-acquired pneumonias, which are usually Gram-positive.

Hospitalization itself causes a change in endogenous bacteria to predominantly Gram-negative pathogens.

Many factors control bacterial virulence. These include resistance to complement, antiphagocytic surfaces (encapsulation), the ability to survive intracellularly, and the ability of some bacteria to produce tissue-toxic enzymes and various exotoxins. The host's defense mechanisms may be violated and weakened and thus allow pathogenic bacteria to cause infection. The skin, for example, is a natural mechanical barrier to infection. This is disturbed with wounding or thermal injury. The nasopharyngeal barrier to pulmonary infection is abolished with endotracheal intubation or tracheostomy. Aspiration is

The use of various tubes and catheters can break down natural host defense.

a common cause of nosocomial pneumonia. A nasogastric tube may contribute to this. Urinary tract infection may occur following catheterization with a Foley catheter, suprapubic tube, or nephrostomy tube. Vascular catheters may also be the source of sepsis. These include routine intravenous lines, arterial lines, central venous pressure (CVP) lines, and Swan-Ganz catheters. Chronic disease, old age, trauma, malnutrition, radiation therapy, and chemotherapy (including the use of corticosteroids) can all cause immunosuppression and thus increase the risk of infection and sepsis.

Patients with chronic disease, old age, and immunosuppression are at increased risk of infection and sepsis.

The incidence of Gram-negative bacteremia in the United States is 100,000–300,000 cases per year. The mortality risk of Gram-negative bacteremia is 20–50%. About 20% of patients with Gram-negative bacteremia will develop septic shock. Septic shock caused by Gram-negative bacteremia carries a 50–80% mortality risk. Most cases of Gram-negative bacteremias are caused by a single organism. However, about 10% of these infections are polymicrobial.

There are 100,000–300,000 cases per year of Gram-negative bacteremia. About 20% of these patients will develop septic shock. This carries a 50–80% mortality risk.

The incidence of Gram-positive bacteremia, on the other hand, is less, about 25,000–50,000 cases per year. Only about 5% of these patients develop septic shock.

About 70% of all cases of Gram-negative bacteremia are acquired in the hospital. The urinary tract is the most common source of the infection. Urinary sepsis is usually preceded by either urinary tract instrumentation with catheters or cystoscopy, or by urinary tract surgery. *Escherichia coli, Klebsiella, Enterobacter, Serratia* species, *Proteus* species, and *Pseudomonas aeruginosa* are the most common causes of infection. Hospital-acquired pneumonia is the second most common infection and is usually caused by *E. coli, Pseudomonas, Klebsiella, Enterobacter, Serratia,* and sometimes *Bacteroides* species. The gastrointestinal tract is the third most common source of infection and accounts for about 20–25% of all cases of Gram-negative bacteremias. Sepsis may result from biliary tract infection (cholecystitis, cholangitis), from bowel obstruction or perforation, from peritonitis, and from intra-abdominal abscesses. The most common organisms are *E. coli, Klebsiella, Enterobacter, Serratia, Bacteroides,* and occasionally *Salmonella.*

About 70% of all cases of Gram-negative bacteremia are acquired in the hospital.

The urinary tract is the most common site of infection. The lungs are the second most common site, and the gastrointestinal tract is the third.

TABLE 5.1   Most Common Agents in Bacterial Sepsis

Agent	Relative Frequency (%)
Gram-positive sepsis	
Staphylococcus aureus	40
Streptococcus pneumoniae	20–25
Group D Streptococcus	10–15
Viridans group of Streptococcus	5–7
Neither group A nor D Streptococcus	5–10
Group A Streptococcus	5
Gram-negative sepsis	
E. coli	40–45
Klebsiella, Enterobacter	20
Pseudomonas aeruginosa	10–15
Bacteroides	10
Proteus	5–7
Serratia	5–7
Haemophilus	2–3
Providencia, Citrobacter	2

Adapted with permission from Youmans GP, Paterson PY, Sommers HM (eds), The Biologic and Clinical Basis of Infectious Disease, W. B. Saunders, Philadelphia, 1980, p 475.

Other potential sources of infection include the skin and wounds, the heart (endocarditis), the brain (abscess, meningitis), bone (osteomyelitis), female pelvic organs (pelvic inflammatory disease, tubo-ovarian abscess, septic abortion, endometritis), and vascular catheters.

The family Enterobacteriaceae causes most cases of septic shock.

The bacterial family Enterobacteriaceae causes most cases of septic shock. Included in this family or organisms are E. coli, Klebsiella, Enterobacter, Serratia, Proteus, Providencia, Arizona, Citrobacter, Hafnia, Salmonella, and Shigella. Table 5.1 lists the most common agents in Gram-positive and Gram-negative bacterial sepsis and their relative frequency of occurrence. Table 5.2 lists the usual sites of infection and the suspected bacteriology.

▨ Diagnosis

The diagnosis of septic shock is usually straightforward. The antecedent history and clinical setting are

TABLE 5.2 Sites of Infection and Suspected Bacteriology

Site	Common Pathogen
Urine	Enterobacteriaceae
	Pseudomonas
	Streptococcus group D enterococcus
Bile	E. coli
	Klebsiella
	Streptococcus group D enterococcus
Intra-abdominal abscess, peritonitis	Enterobacteriaceae
	Bacteroides
Pneumonia (nosocomial)	Enterobacteriaceae
	Staphylococcus aureus
	Anaerobes
Female genital tract	Enterobacteriaceae
	Bacteroides
	Clostridia
	Anaerobic Gram-positive cocci
Decubiti	Enterobacteriaceae
	Staphylococcus aureus
	Pseudomonas
	Bacteroides
Intravenous catheters	Enterobacteriaceae
	Staphylococcus aureus

Adapted with permission from Landesman SH, Gorbach SL. Gram-negative sepsis and shock. Orthop Clin North Am 9:617, 1978.

important. Certain groups of patients are known to be at increased risk of developing clinical sepsis. At high risk are the elderly, the premature newborn, and those with chronic diseases such as diabetes, cirrhosis, and malnutrition. Patients with leukemia, lymphoma, and other malignancies receiving chemotherapy or radiation therapy are at high risk. Surgery or instrumentation of the urinary tract, the biliary tract, or the gastrointestinal tract all predispose to the development of bacterial sepsis. The postsplenectomy patient is also at risk. The female patient who undergoes an incomplete abortion, a cesarean section, or hysterectomy for pelvic inflammatory disease is at increased risk. Patients with primary immunodeficiency disorders are at high risk. Childbirth, trauma, burn injury, and the use of broad-spectrum antibiotics can all predispose the patient to Gram-negative sepsis. *(Patients at increased risk of becoming septic)*

Most patients with septic shock present with fever (above 101°F), chills, and hypotension. In Gram- *(Most septic patients are febrile.)*

Hypothermia can occur particularly in the newborn or elderly patient.

Hyperventilation and an altered mental status are early signs of sepsis.

Any hospitalized patient who develops fever, chills, hyperventilation, and an altered mental status should be considered septic.

The two major clinical syndromes of bacterial septic shock are warm shock and cold shock.

Cold shock is a more severe form than warm shock.

negative bacterial sepsis about 60% of patients will have chills and fever. Another 25% will have spiking fever without chills. Some patients will develop fever gradually in association with general malaise. Occasionally hypothermia will be noted. This is particularly true for the geriatric patient or the premature newborn.

Two of the earliest manifestations of bacterial sepsis are hyperventilation and changes in mental status. The hyperventilation may result from a direct effect of bacterial endotoxin on the medullary respiratory center. The resulting respiratory alkalosis is thus an early sign of Gram-negative bacterial sepsis. The patient's sensorium may be altered and cause confusion, lethargy, stupor, and, on occasion, even coma.

From the above it is clear that the diagnosis of bacterial sepsis should be strongly considered in any patient who develops fever, chills, hyperventilation, and altered mental status. This is particularly true for the hospitalized patient with known predisposing factors for the development of sepsis. The institution of therapy during this early stage of clinical sepsis before the development of hemodynamic instability may be life-saving.

In humans there are two major clinical syndromes of bacterial septic shock. The minority of patients present with warm, dry, pink skin, adequate urine output, and normal mental status despite hypotension. This warm shock syndrome results from peripheral vasodilatation and/or arteriovenous shunting. Septic shock caused by Gram-positive organisms and fungi are usually of the warm shock type, at least initially.

The majority of patients, however, present with cold, moist skin, hypotension, oliguria, peripheral cyanosis, and altered sensorium. Many of the manifestations of this cold shock syndrome are due to intense vasoconstriction. Septic shock caused by Gram-negative organisms can be of either the warm or the cold shock type. This progression is the clinical manifestation of increasing circulatory insufficiency.

Cold shock is a more severe form of shock than warm shock. Whether or not a patient presents initially with warm or cold shock depends on the type of infecting organism, the initial volume status of the patient, and the patient's homeostatic defense capabilities. The pathophysiology of these two clinical pictures of septic shock will be discussed in detail in the next section, "Pathophysiology."

Skin lesions can occur in sepsis and septic shock. The lesions of ecthyma gangrenosum occur in 5–25% of all cases of *Pseudomonas aeruginosa* bacteremia. They may also be found in *Aeromonas hydrophila* bacteremia. These lesions consist of a necrotic center surrounded by an area of erythema and are located most commonly in the axilla and anogenital areas. Skin lesions can also be found in sepsis due to *E. coli, Klebsiella, Enterobacter,* and *Serratia* and include bullae, vesicles, areas of cellulitis or erythema, and petechiae.

Other findings in sepsis and septic shock may include pulmonary insufficiency and the adult respiratory distress syndrome. Hypoxemia may be severe. Renal insufficiency may develop, causing oliguria or anuria. Occasionally high-output acute renal failure will occur. Sepsis and septic shock can also cause hepatic dysfunction and jaundice. The hemodynamic alterations in septic shock are variable. The cardiac index may be normal, increased, or decreased. The heart rate may be normal, increased, or decreased. Thrombocytopenia may occur, and on occasion sepsis may induce a disseminated intravascular coagulation (DIC) syndrome. Acute gastric erosion and gastrointestinal hemorrhage may complicate sepsis and shock. Leukopenia or leukocytosis may be found. In general, there is a shift to immature white blood cell forms on differential count. Acid-base derangements occur. As stated before, there may be an initial respiratory alkalosis due to hyperventilation. As shock progresses, however, the accumulation of lactic acid and subsequent lactic acidemia causes a metabolic acidosis. Table 5.3 outlines the major clinical findings in sepsis and septic shock.

Once the diagnosis of clinical sepsis is made, blood cultures should be obtained. Cultures should also be taken from probable sites of infection, namely, urine, sputum, wound, etc. Ideally cultures should be obtained prior to the institution of antibiotic therapy. Three sets of blood cultures are recommended. In about 80% of cases with proven bacteremia the

Which shock picture predominates depends on the infecting pathogen, the volume status of the patient, and the patient's defense mechanisms.

Skin lesions may occur in sepsis.

The clinical findings in sepsis are variable.

Three sets of blood cultures should be obtained.

TABLE 5.3   Findings in Sepsis and Septic Shock

Fever	Bleeding disorder
Hypothermia	Thrombocytopenia
Chills	DIC syndrome
Hypotension	Leukocytosis
Hyperventilation	Leukopenia
Altered mental status	Hypoxemia
Skin lesions	Respiratory alkalosis
Tachycardia	Metabolic acidosis
Bradycardia	Oliguria
Normal, high, or low cardiac output	Jaundice

first set of blood cultures will be positive. The positivity rate approaches 98% by the third set. Three days of incubation and three sets of blood cultures accurately identify over 90% of all Gram-negative bacteremias. For patients already on antibiotic treatment when sepsis occurs, the blood cultures should be observed in incubation for 10 days. Sometimes blood cultures remain negative when bacteremias are intermittent. Negative cultures, therefore, do not necessarily rule out bacteremia. The patient should be treated for sepsis if the clinical state supports the diagnosis, regardless of culture results. Apart from blood cultures there exists no other laboratory test that is specific for the diagnosis of sepsis.

Negative blood cultures do not rule out bacteremia.

Pathophysiology

The pathophysiology of sepsis and septic shock is complex and only partially understood. The basic cause for the circulatory insufficiency that may complicate sepsis is unknown. There is some recent evidence to implicate various endogenous opiate compounds, called endorphins, in the pathogenesis of septic shock. The experimental administration of naloxone, an opiate antagonist, corrects some of the hemodynamic dysfunction found in endotoxin shock. The exact role of endorphins in septic shock remains to be proven.

Endorphins may play a role in the pathogenesis of septic shock.

There is much data to support the theory that endotoxin is responsible for many of the pathophysiologic abnormalities of Gram-negative septic shock. The outer membrane of the cell wall of the Gram-

Endotoxin causes many of the changes noted in Gram-negative septic shock.

negative bacillus is composed of a lipopolysac-
charide. The polysaccharide moiety of the outer
membrane confers type O somatic antigenicity to the
bacterium. The lipid A moiety of the outer membrane, on the other hand, is responsible for the endotoxic activity of Gram-negative bacteria. Endotoxin (lipid A) is released during lysis of the bacterial
cell wall. Experimental administration of endotoxin
reproduces many of the pathophysiologic changes
seen in humans during Gram-negative sepsis.

When discussing the role of endotoxin in the
pathogenesis of septic shock, however, two points
need emphasis. First, there are some differences in
the hemodynamic sequelae of endotoxin infusion and
live bacteria infusion in the experimental model.
Second, the endotoxin theory does not explain the
pathogenesis of septic shock in Gram-positive bacteremia or sepsis caused by fungus, parasites, viruses, and rickettsia. Nonetheless, the endotoxin
theory has strong support, at least in Gram-negative
sepsis.

A word of caution about the endotoxin theory

The pathophysiologic effects of endotoxin are
numerous (Figure 5.1). Endotoxin can cause fever
both by a direct effect on the thermoregulatory center
of the hypothalamus and by a stimulating effect on
leukocytes to produce endogenous pyrogen. Endotoxin has four major humoral effects. It can activate
the complement system, the coagulation system, the
plasmin-fibrinolysin system, and the kinin system.

Endotoxin has many effects.

Endotoxin can activate the complement cascade by four means: 1) via the classic pathway,
2) via the alternative (properdin) pathway, 3) via a
direct effect on complement factor C1, and 4) via
activation of Hageman factor (factor XII) of the coagulation system. Overall, complement activation
enhances the inflammatory response and is an important homeostatic defense mechanism against infection. The main effects of the complement cascade
include: 1) the ability to damage bacterial cell membranes and cause bacteriolysis (via factors C8 and
C9), 2) the ability to increase capillary permeability
(via factors C3a and C5a, which are also called anaphylatoxins), 3) chemotaxis of polymorphonuclear
leukocytes to sites of infection (via factors C5a, C3a
[?], and activated C5b-6-7), and 4) enhancement of
phagocytosis by polymorphonuclear leukocytes (via

Endotoxin activates the complement cas-cade by four means.

The effects of comple-ment activation are several. In general, the complement cascade enhances the inflam-matory response.

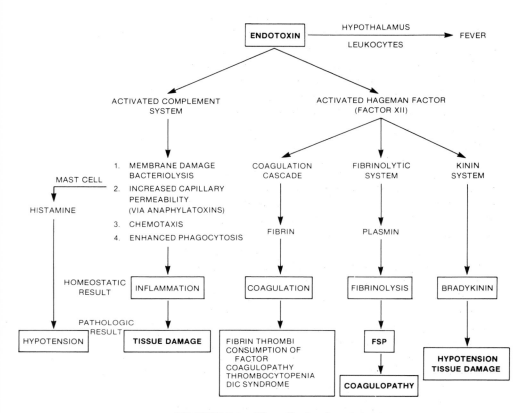

FIGURE 5.1   The effects of endotoxin are numerous. Endotoxin can activate the complement system, the coagulation system, the plasmin-fibrinolytic system, and the kinin system. The effects of these systems are to cause hypotension, tissue damage, and a consumptive coagulopathy. Adapted with permission from Gleckman R, Esposito A. Gram-negative bacteremic shock: Pathophysiologic clinical features and treatment. South Med J 74:337, 1981; and Mandell GL, Douglas RG Jr, Bennett JE (eds), Principles and Practice of Infectious Diseases. John Wiley, New York, 1979, p 584.

Endotoxin can also activate the coagulation system, the plasmin-fibrinolysin system, and the kinin system.

factors C3b and C5b). It should be noted that the anaphylatoxins (factors C3a and C5a) can also induce tissue mast cells to release histamine, which in turn causes vasodilation of blood vessels.

Endotoxin can also activate the Hageman factor (factor XII) of the coagulation system. Activated Hageman factor then initiates the coagulation cascade, the plasmin-fibrinolysin system, and the kinin system. The coagulation cascade causes the ultimate deposition of fibrin and thrombosis. Activation of the fibrinolysin system causes fibrin degeneration and the production of fibrin split products. Likewise, activation of the kinin system causes production of bradykinin. Bradykinin can increase capillary permeability and cause vasodilation of blood vessels.

The body's humoral responses to endotoxin, namely, activiation of the complement, coagulation, fibrinolysin, and kinin systems, all play an important role in normal homeostasis against infection. Complement activation results in an enhanced inflammatory response. Capillary permeability is increased by anaphylatoxins, histamine, and bradykinin. The generation of plasmin (fibrinolysin) acts as a check and balance against excessive thrombosis. However, during sepsis and septic shock the biologic effects of endotoxin activation of the above-mentioned systems may become pathologic. Complement activation enhances the inflammatory response. This may cause further tissue damage and increase capillary permeability, resulting in the release of lysosomal enzymes (which are cytotoxic) and a loss of effective blood volume. Fibrin deposition and thrombosis may cause tissue ischemia and further tissue necrosis. The consumption of clotting factors and platelets during the coagulation cascade may result in thrombocytopenia and coagulopathy with hemorrhaging. A DIC syndrome may result. Fibrinolysis causes the production of fibrin split products. There protein fragments function as anticoagulants and can therefore enhance the coagulopathy. Finally, histamine and bradykinin cause vasodilation and can lower total peripheral resistance, resulting in systemic hypotension.

The biologic effects of endotoxin may become pathologic and cause tissue damage, hypotension, and a consumptive coagulopathy.

As stated earlier, there are two major clinical syndromes of septic shock. Warm shock (or early shock) is characterized by a normal or elevated cardiac output and a lowered total peripheral resistance. The altered peripheral resistance in this form may result from bradykinin and histamine production as well as the peripheral shunting of blood through lower resistance arteriovenous anastomosis. Cold shock (or late shock) is characterized by a decreased cardiac output and an increased total peripheral resistance. In this form of septic shock the peripheral vessels are markedly vasoconstricted be-

In warm shock the cardiac output is normal or high and the peripheral resistance is low.

In cold shock the cardiac output is low and the peripheral resistance is high.

Cold shock is the clinical manifestation of severe circulatory failure.

cause of a major adrenergic response (via catecholamine and neurogenic influences). Cold shock is the clinical manifestation of severe circulatory insufficiency.

Clinically, one should view septic shock as a continuous spectrum between the warm and cold types. Some patients pass from the warm (early) septic shock to cold (late) septic shock. Other patients present initially in cold shock. Hypotension, by definition, is common to both warm and cold shock. The specific hemodynamic profile of each septic patient depends to a large degree on the preseptic volume status of the patient as well as the patient's myocardial reserve. For example, a well hydrated young adult would most commonly present initially with warm shock when septic. If left untreated this young patient would progress into cold shock as circulatory insufficiency became worse. Likewise, a dehydrated geriatric patient with known coronary artery disease would most commonly present initially with cold shock. The cold shock syndrome is seen most commonly, moreover, when the intravascular blood volume has been depleted by third space losses, as in peritonitis with sepsis.

The preseptic volume status and the myocardial reserve are important considerations.

The hemodynamic profiles of warm and cold shock can be displayed graphically.

The hemodynamic alterations of warm and cold septic shock can be viewed graphically via the systemic and ventricular function curves. In warm shock the total peripheral resistance is decreased (Figure 5.2). This causes a reduction in afterload. The systemic function curve rotates clockwise, and the ventricular function curve shifts upward and to the left. The resultant equilibrium point (point B) represents a hyperdynamic state in which cardiac output is improved for the same level of ventricular preload. Upon initial view it seems somewhat paradoxical that this improved cardiac performance is accompanied by hypotension. It should be recalled, however, that blood pressure is directly proportional to the product of cardiac output and total peripheral resistance. In warm shock, therefore, the hemodynamic effects of sepsis cause a decrease in the resistance factor greater than the increase in the cardiac output factor. The result is systemic hypotension.

Warm shock causes a hyperdynamic state.

In cold shock the total peripheral resistance is increased due to adrenergic stimulation (Figure 5.3). This causes an increase in the afterload. The sys-

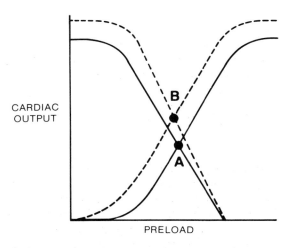

CARDIAC OUTPUT

PRELOAD

FIGURE 5.2 Warm septic shock is characterized by a normal or an elevated cardiac output and a lowered total peripheral vascular resistance. The systemic function curve rotates clockwise (due to decreased afterload), and the ventricular function curve shifts upward and to the left (due to improved contractility and afterload reduction). The new equilibrium point (B) represents improved cardiac performance. Clinically, however, the patient may be hypotensive because of the major effect of lowered vascular resistance on blood pressure.

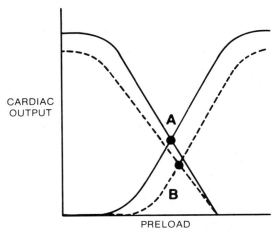

CARDIAC OUTPUT

PRELOAD

FIGURE 5.3 Cold septic shock is characterized by a decreased cardiac output and an elevated total peripheral resistance. The systemic function curve rotates counterclockwise (due to increased afterload), and the ventricular function curve shifts downward and to the right (due to decreased contractility and increased afterload). The new equilibrium point (B) represents failing cardiac performance.

temic function curve rotates counterclockwise, and the ventricular function curve shifts downward and to the right. The new equilibrium point (point B) represents a hypodynamic state. Cardiac output is lowered for each level of ventricular preload. The exact mechanism for poor cardiac performance during cold septic shock is not known. Increasing afterload certainly plays a role. Other potential factors in its pathogenesis include the effects of increasing metabolic acidemia on the myocardium, coronary artery disease and poor myocardial perfusion, and the influence of humoral factors such as the myocardial depressant factor.

Cold shock causes a hypodynamic state.

The cause of poor cardiac performance in cold septic shock is multifactorial.

In septic shock the hemodynamic mechanism is primarily one of altered vascular resistance. It is clear from the above that alterations in blood volume and in cardiac output also play a role in its pathogenesis.

In hemorrhagic and cardiogenic shock there is a decreased cardiac output associated with an increased arteriovenous O_2 difference. An increased arteriovenous O_2 difference implies that the tissues are using more O_2. In septic shock, however, there is a defect in O_2 utilization by the peripheral tissues. In sepsis the arteriovenous O_2 difference is actually lowered, meaning that the tissues are using less O_2. This lack of cellular O_2 utilization may be the prime defect in septic shock that ultimately leads to cellular failure and death. The details of this important abnormality are unknown at present but may be due to a mitochondrial malfunction.

In sepsis there is a defect in O_2 utilization by tissues. Why this occurs is unknown.

Treatment

The overall mortality rate of Gram-negative septic shock is about 50% despite all known modalities of medical and surgical therapy. The optimal treatment, therefore, obviously involves prevention of shock during sepsis. The physician at all times must remain keenly cognizant of the predisposing risk factors in sepsis, the clinical setting in which sepsis might occur, and the actual signs and symptoms of septic shock. Delay in treatment may have an irreversible and fatal outcome.

Optimal therapy involves preventing shock during sepsis.

The treatment of sepsis and septic shock involves six avenues of therapy: 1) support of the respiratory system, 2) treatment of infection, 3) support of the cardiovascular system, 4) corticosteroids, 5) establishment of normothermia, and 6) treatment of clotting dysfunction.

Regardless of the cause of shock, an adequate airway must be secured if resuscitative efforts are to be successful. Rapid assessment of airway function is essential in the initial treatment of septic shock. If respiratory distress is present, the patient must be intubated immediately and ventilated artificially with 100% oxygen. Most patients with sepsis can be managed initially with oxygen administered via mask or nasal prong. Respiratory function can then be assessed further with arterial blood gas analysis. If the airway is in doubt or the ventilatory function of the patient is questionable, it is better to establish a definite airway and subsequently remove it rather than to procrastinate and allow the possibility for respiratory arrest.

The first priority is to secure adequate respiratory function.

Treatment of infection does not only include the use of antimicrobial agents. More importantly, the cause of infection must be ascertained and treated promptly. Antibiotics should play an ancillary role only, and total reliance on their potential efficacy should be avoided. Surgical intervention may be required. This may involve drainage of intra-abdominal abscesses, resection of ischemic and necrotic bowel, cholecystectomy, common bile duct exploration, tube thoracostomy in thoracic empyema, and the like, depending on the specific etiologic focus. The timing of surgical operation in the treatment of sepsis from intra-abdominal causes is beyond the scope of this book. In general, however, with newly diagnosed intra-abdominal sepsis the patient should be treated medically initially for at least a few hours in order to reestablish a more euvolemic state and to correct any existing electrolyte or anemic disorder prior to general anesthesia. This delay in surgical intervention is required so as to optimize the patient's overall condition prior to surgery. Astute preoperative preparation is essential.

The cause of infection should be promptly determined.

Antibiotics play an ancillary role in the treatment of sepsis.

Surgery may be needed.

There are numerous antibiotics available to the physician. Table 5.4 lists the antibiotics of choice for most causes of sepsis. Table 5.5 lists the dosage

TABLE 5.4   Choice of Antibiotics in Sepsis

Pathogen	Drug of Choice	Alternatives
Gram-positive bacteria		
Staphylococcus aureus	Oxacillin	Cephalosporin Vancomycin
Streptococcus pneumoniae	Penicillin G	Cephalosporin Erythromycin
Group D Streptococcus enterococcus	Ampicillin with gentamicin	Vancomycin with gentamicin
Streptococcus viridans	Penicillin G with or without streptomycin	Cephalosporin Vancomycin
Streptococcus pyogenes	Penicillin G	Cephalosporin Erythromycin
Clostridium	Penicillin G	Cephalosporin Erythromycin
Anaerobic Streptococcus	Penicillin G	Cephalosporin Erythromycin Clindamycin
Gram-negative bacteria		
E. coli	Gentamicin or tobramycin	Ampicillin Amikacin Cephalosporin Chloramphenicol
Klebsiella pneumonia	Gentamicin or tobramycin	Amikacin Cephalosporin Chloramphenicol
Enterobacter	Gentamicin or tobramycin	Amikacin Carbenicillin Ticarcillin Cefamandole Chloramphenicol
Pseudomonas aeruginosa	Gentamicin or tobramycin with or without carbenicillin or ticarcillin	Amikacin
Bacteroides, respiratory	Penicillin G	Clindamycin Chloramphenicol
Bacteroides, gastrointestinal	Clindamycin	Metronidazole Cefoxitin Chloramphenicol
Proteus mirabilis	Ampicillin	Cephalosporin Gentamicin Tobramycin Amikacin Carbenicillin Ticarcillin, chloramphenicol

TABLE 5.4   Choice of Antibiotics in Sepsis (*Continued*)

Pathogen	Drug of Choice	Alternatives
Proteus, other	Gentamicin or tobramycin	Cephalosporin Amikacin Carbenicillin or ticarcillin Cefoxitin Chloramphenicol
Serratia marcescens	Gentamicin or tobramycin	Amikacin Cefoxitin Carbenicillin or ticarcillin Chloramphenicol
Haemophilus influenzae life-threatening other infection	Chloramphenicol Ampicillin	Ampicillin Chloramphenicol Cefamandole
Salmonella typhi	Chloramphenicol	Ampicillin Trimethoprim- sulfamethoxazole
Shigella	Ampicillin	Trimethoprim- sulfamethoxazole Chloramphenicol
Providencia	Amikacin	Gentamicin or tobramycin Carbenicillin or ticarcillin Cefamandole or cefoxitin Chloramphenicol
Citrobacter freundii	Gentamicin or tobramycin	Chloramphenicol Carbenicillin
Acinetobacter (also *Mima, Herellea*)	Gentamicin or tobramycin	Amikacin

In sepsis of unknown etiology, use ampicillin or oxacillin or cephalosporin with gentamicin or tobramycin.

If anaerobes are expected, add clindamycin or chloramphenicol or metronidazole.

Adapted with permission from Abramowitz M (ed), The choice of antimicrobial drugs. The Medical Letter 22:8, 1980.

schedule for these antibiotics along with a compilation of their more common adverse effects. Antibiotics should be administered intravenously in sepsis so as to assure adequate blood levels.

In septic shock of unknown etiology it is important to start antibiotics that will cover both Gram-positive and Gram-negative bacteria. This involves combining two antibiotics. A penicillinase-resistant penicillin (oxacillin) or a cephalosporin should be combined with an aminoglycoside (gentamicin or to-

Antibiotic choice in sepsis of unknown etiology

TABLE 5.5   **Dosage Schedule for Antimicrobial Agents (for Adults)**

Agent	Dose (IV)	Possible Adverse Effects
Penicillins		
Penicillin G	1–5 million units q4–6h	Allergic reaction
		Anaphylactic shock
Oxacillin	0.5–2 g q4–6h	
Ampicillin	0.5–2 g q4–6h	Diarrhea
		Pseudomembranous colitis
Carbenicillin	20–40 g/day in 6 doses	Sodium overload
		Platelet dysfunction
		Hemorrhagic cystitis
Ticarcillin	12–24 g/day in 6 doses	Sodium overload
		Platelet dysfunction
Cephalosporins		
Cephalothin	1–2 g q4–6h	Allergic reaction
Cephapirin	1–2 g q4–6h	Thrombophlebitis
Cefazolin	0.5–1 g q4–8h	Pseudomembranous colitis
Cefamandole	1–2 g q4–6h	
Cefoxitin	1–2 g q4–8h	
Cefotaxime	1–2 g q4–8h	
Aminoglycosides		
Gentamicin	1–2 mg/kg q8h	Vestibular-auditory damage
Tobramycin	1–2 mg/kg q8h	Renal damage
Amikacin	15 mg/kg/day in 2–3 doses	
Streptomycin	0.5–1 g q12h	
Other		
Chloramphenicol	0.5–1.0 g q6h	Gray syndrome in infants
		Aplastic anemia
		Pseudomembranous colitis
		Blood dyscrasias
Clindamycin	0.3–0.6 g q6h	Diarrhea
		Pseudomembranous colitis
Metronidazole	15 mg/kg (1 g) loading dose	Seizures
	7.5 mg/kg (0.5 g) q6h	Peripheral neuropathy
Vancomycin	0.5 g q6h	Thrombophlebitis
		Renal damage
		Eighth-nerve damage
Erythromycin	0.5–1.0 g q6h	Cholestatic hepatitis
		Stomatitis
		Pseudomembranous colitis
Trimethoprim-	2 tabs po q12h	Allergy
Sulfamethoxazole		Steven-Johnson snydrome
		Blood dyscrasias
		Renal damage
		Liver damage
		Pseudomembranous colitis

Adapted with permission from Freitag JJ, Miller LW (eds), Manual of Medical Therapeutics, 23rd ed. Little, Brown, Boston, 1980, p 178; Harvey HM, Johns RJ, McKusick VA, et al. (eds), The Principles and Practice of Medicine, 20th ed. Appleton-Century-Crofts, New York, 1980, pp 945, 949; Abramowitz M (ed), Adverse effects of antimicrobial drugs, Handbook of Antimicrobial Therapy. The Medical Letter, New Rochelle NY, 1980, p. 29.

braymycin). Empiric therapy with this combination will be effective against most cases of sepsis due to the Enterobacteriaceae, *Pseudomonas aeruginosa*, and *Staphylococcus aureus*. Some physicians will use ampicillin combined with an aminoglycoside so as to treat possible group D streptococcal (enterococcus) sepsis. This is particularly true when the source of infection is probably either the urinary or the biliary tract. If an anaerobic infection is suspected, as in bowel perforation or pelvic inflammatory disease, then either clindamycin, chloramphenicol, carbenicillin, metronidazole, or cefoxitin should be added. *Pseudomonas* sepsis is common in the burn patient and the leukemic patient who develops sepsis. In this setting carbenicillin may be combined with an aminoglycoside until culture results become available. Once the specific pathogen is identified, then the antibiotic regimen can be made more specific and less broad-spectrum.

Support of the cardiovascular system in septic shock involves: 1) reestablishing normovolemia and 2) improving cardiac performance. These two functions are interrelated because of the influence of blood volume on the ventricular preload and cardiac output.

Most patients in septic shock are hypovolemic. This is particularly true for those clinical states associated with large third space fluid losses, as in peritonitis, strangulated bowel obstruction, and burn injury. It is important to establish appropriate monitoring devices early in the course of sepsis. An arterial line should be inserted so as to measure continuous blood pressure. A Foley catheter should be inserted to measure hourly urine output. Following urine output is a simple way to monitor organ (kidney) perfusion. A CVP or Swan-Ganz catheter should be placed so as to assess the volume status and preload state of the heart. The Swan-Ganz catheter is preferred when there is coexisting pulmonary, cardiac, or renal insufficiency.

The object of fluid resuscitation in septic shock is to reestablish normovolemia and to optimize the ventricular preload. The intravenous infusion of crystalloid solution (either lactated Ringer's or normal saline) is used for this purpose. CVP or pul-

Antibiotic choice in anaerobic infection

Cardiovascular support involves establishing normovolemia and improving cardiac performance.

Insert monitoring devices early in sepsis.

Establishing normovolemia optimizes the ventricular preload.

monary capillary wedge pressure (PCWP) can be used as a guide to fluid therapy. Volume is administered until the horizontal phase of the cardiac function curve is attained.

CVP or PCWP should be used to guide fluid therapy.

If the initial CVP or PCWP is low, bolus therapy using crystalloid solution is warranted. From 200 to 250 ml of normal saline or lactated Ringer's can be administered rapidly. If the CVP or PCWP fails to rise after 10–15 minutes, the bolus may be repeated as needed. If a 200 to 250-ml fluid bolus markedly elevates the CVP or PCWP without improving the overall hemodynamic profile, then the patient may be in borderline fluid overload and bolus therapy should be discontinued. Bolus therapy should also be curtailed if the CVP reaches 12–15 cm H_2O or the PCWP reaches 15–18 mm Hg.

Transfusion therapy may be required.

If the septic patient is hypovolemic and anemic, blood in the form of packed red blood cells should be administered as a volume-loading agent in addition to crystalloid solution. If the septic patient is hypovolemic and has a coagulopathy, fresh frozen plasma (FFP) can be given as a volume agent.

Albumin should be avoided.

Albumin should be avoided unless salt must be restricted (as in the cirrhotic with ascites) or the patient is markedly hypoproteinemic. There is little role for albumin therapy in septic shock except under these two circumstances.

If septic shock remains refractory to volume loading, then therapy should be directed at the heart and the peripheral vessels. The patient should be given intravenous digoxin so as to improve the inotropic state of the myocardium. In addition, an infusion of dopamine should be started. This agent

Dopamine is the drug of choice in the treatment of shock refractory to volume loading.

should be the initial sympathomimetic amine used in the treatment of septic shock refractory to volume loading. Inotropic and vasoactive agents can be used if dopamine is unsuccessful in improving the hemodynamic profile. These agents include dobutamine, isoproterenol, norepinephrine, and epinephrine. The reader is referred to the section on "Treatment," in Chapter 2, for a detailed review of the pharmacology of these agents.

As stated earlier, some patients present initially in warm shock (normal or high cardiac output, decreased peripheral resistance) and then may deteriorate over time into cold shock (decreased cardiac output, increased peripheral resistance). On a theoretical basis norepinephrine or phenylephrine would seem a good choice as a vasopressor agent in warm shock because of their ability to cause vasoconstriction. Although blood pressure would increase with its use, perfusion at the microcirculatory level would decrease and tissue ischemia would be made worse.

In cold shock, however, there is marked peripheral vasoconstriction. In cold shock, if the circulation has adequate volume and if shock remains refractory to inotropic support (digoxin, dopamine), then there is justification for the use of afterload-reducing agents such as nitroprusside. The combination of dopamine and nitroprusside in this setting may substantially improve the hemodynamic profile of the patient.

Cardiac performance may improve by the combined use of dopamine and nitroprusside in cold shock.

Steroids seem to be beneficial in the treatment of septic shock, although the literature is controversial. Most physicians use steroids in septic shock, not only to treat the sepsis but also to protect against the possibility of adrenal insufficiency. A bolus dose of methylprednisolone 30 mg/kg IV is given acutely and every 4 hours as needed for 24–48 hours. This is discussed further in Chapter 2 under "Treatment."

The febrile patient in septic shock should be treated with acetaminophen (10–20 grains) as a rectal suppository every 4 hours as needed. Alcohol sponge baths and a cooling blanket may be needed. Conversely, the hypothermic patient should be treated with a heating blanket.

Control body temperature.

Sepsis can cause activation of both the clotting and the fibrinolytic systems. The prothrombin time may become prolonged. This should be treated with vitamin K injections and by FFP infusions. Thrombocytopenia should be corrected with platelet transfusions if the platelet count decreases to less than 50,000 in the bleeding septic patient. Occasionally a DIC syndrome occurs. This can be diagnosed by measuring levels of fibrinogen and fibrin split products. The best treatment for the DIC syndrome in sepsis is to treat the focus of infection. Occasionally heparin may be needed, although its use is controversial.

Case Study

A 60-year-old man undergoes an elective inguinal hernia repair. His postoperative course is unremarkable except for urinary retention, which requires a Foley catheter for 4 days. The nurses report that he is confused on the fifth postoperative day. On exam he appears in no acute distress, BP and pulse are normal, but respiratory rate is 30. He is afebrile. His wound is clean. He is somewhat confused and cannot remember the date. The nurses are instructed to keep a close eye on him. About 2 hours later the nurses call and say that his BP is now 75 mm Hg. On exam he is confused and agitated and has cold, moist extremities. He has no specific complaints. BP is 75 mm Hg, pulse rate 120, and respiratory rate is 35. Only 120 ml of urine is noted for the previous 8 hours. A peripheral IV is started with normal saline wide open, a CVP line is inserted and measures 2 cm H_2O, blood work and an ABG are drawn, 40% O_2 is given by mask, and an EKG is obtained stat and reveals only sinus tachycardia. A stat portable chest x-ray is unremarkable. The ABG reveals $PO_2 = 95$ mm Hg, $PCO_2 = 25$ mm Hg, and pH 7.38. The white blood cell count is 11,000 with 60 polys and 22 bands. Blood cultures are drawn, a urinalysis is sent stat, and a urine culture is obtained.

Ampicillin 2 g and gentamicin 80 mg are given intravenously. One liter of saline is administered over 20 min. The BP is now 90 mm Hg and the CVP is 6 cm H_2O. A bolus dose of 2 g methylprednisolone is give intravenously. Another liter of saline is given over 20 min. The BP is now 95 mm Hg and the CVP is 8 cm H_2O. Dopamine (10 µg/kg/min) infusion is started. The BP increases to 120 mm Hg. The patient is transferred to the intensive care unit for further care. The urinalysis reveals 50 white blood cells per field with loaded bacteria. The next day the bacteriology lab reports that both the blood and urine cultures are positive for Gram-negative rods.

The above case illustrates a common clinical problem, namely, iatrogenic urosepsis secondary to an indwelling urinary catheter. Points that should be noted include: 1) the initial mental confusion with tachypnea should have been a clue for possible early sepsis in this clinical setting; 2) initial resuscitation involves volume therapy; 3) broad-spectrum antibiotics are begun empirically once the clinical diagnosis of sepsis is made; 4) dopamine can be used judiciously in this setting as volume replacement is being completed; and 5) most physicians would institute a short course of high-dose steroids in the treatment regimen of septic shock.

Annotated Bibliography

Eskridge RA. Septic shock. Crit Care Q 2:55–75, 1980.
A recent review of septic shock and its therapy.

Forgacs P. Treatment of septic shock. Med Clin North Am 63:465–471, 1979.
A concise review on the etiology and treatment of septic shock.

Gleckman R, Esposito A. Gram-negative bacteremic shock: Pathophysiology, clinical features and treatment. South Med J 74:335–341, 1981.
An excellent up-to-date review of the pathophysiology of septic shock.

Landesman SH, Gorbach SL. Gram-negative sepsis and shock. Orthop Clin North Am 9:611–625, 1978.
Reviews the common pathogens for various sites of infection.

Mandell GL, Douglas RG Jr, Bennett JE (ed). Principles and Practice of Infectious Diseases. John Wiley, New York, 1979.
A comprehensive review of Gram-negative bacteremia and septic shock.

Meakins JL, Wirklund BK, Forse RA, et al. The surgical intensive care unit: Current concepts in infection. Surg Clin North Am 60:117–132, 1980.
A detailed review of the epidemiology of nosocomial infection in the intensive care unit.

Schumer W. Steroids in the treatment of clinical septic shock. Ann Surg 184:333–341, 1976.
Schumer's clinical study on the use of steroids in sepsis.

Youmans GP, Paterson PY, Sommers HM (eds). The

Biologic and Clinical Basis of Infectious Disease. W. B. Saunders, Philadelphia, 1980.

A detailed review of Gram-negative bacteremia and sepsis.

Additional Bibliography

Abramowitz M (ed). The choice of antimicrobial drugs. The Medical Letter 22:5–12, 1980.

Abramowitz M (ed). The Medical Letter on Drugs and Therapeutics. The Medical Letter, Inc., New Rochelle NY, 1980.

Baue AE. The treatment of septic shock: A problem intensified by advancing science. Surgery 65:850–859, 1969.

Brachman PS, Dan RB, Haley RW, et al. Nosocomial surgical infections: Incidence and cost. Surg Clin North Am 60:15–25, 1980.

Cavanagh D, Rao PS. Septic shock (endotoxic shock). Clin Obstet Gynecol 16:25–37, 1973.

Christy JH. Pathophysiology of Gram-negative shock. Am Heart J 81:694–701, 1971.

Cruse PJE, Foord R. The epidemiology of wound infection. Surg Clin North Am 60:27–40, 1980.

Davis BD, Dulbecco R, Eisen HN, et al. Microbiology. Harper & Row, New York, 1973.

Duff P. Pathophysiology and management of septic shock. J Reprod Med 24:109–117, 1980.

Esrig BC, Fulton RL. Sepsis, resuscitation, hemorrhagic shock and shock lung. Ann Surg 182:218–227, 1975.

Finegold SM. Anaerobic infections. Surg Clin North Am 60:49–64, 1980.

Freitag JJ, Miller LW (ed). Manual of Medical Therapeutics. Little, Brown, Boston, 1980.

Fulton RL, Jones CE. The cause of post-traumatic pulmonary insufficiency in man. Surg Gynecol Obstet 140:179–186, 1975.

Gelin L, Davidson I, Haglund U, et al. Septic shock. Surg Clin North Am 60:161–174, 1980.

Harvey HM, Johns RJ, McKusick VA, et al. (eds). The Principles and Practice of Medicine. Appleton-Century-Crofts, New York, 1980.

Hassen A. Gram-negative bacteremic shock. Med Clin North Am 57:1403–1415, 1973.

Isselbacher KJ, Adams RD, Braunwald E, et al. (eds). Harrison's Principles of Internal Medicine, 9th ed. McGraw-Hill, New York, 1980, pp. 561–566.

Jawetz E, Melnick JL, Adelberg EA. Review of Medical Microbiology. Lange, Los Altos CA, 1974.

Lucas CE. The real response to acute injury and sepsis. Surg Clin North Am 56:953–975, 1976.

Martin WU. Bacteremia and bacteremic shock in surgical patients. Surg Clin North Am 49:1053–1070, 1969.

Shine KI, Kuhn M, Young LS, et al. Aspects in the management of shock. Ann Intern Med 93:723–734, 1979.

Siegel JH, Cerra FB, Coleman B, et al. Physiological and metabolic correlations in human sepsis. Surgery 86:163–193, 1979.

Weil M. Current understanding of the mechanisms and treatment of circulatory shock caused by bacterial infections. Ann Clin Res 9:181–191, 1977.

Neurogenic Shock 6

Overview

Neurogenic shock is that clinical shock syndrome that results from a decrease in total peripheral vascular resistance. A mismatch between blood volume and vascular capacitance occurs. Common causes of neurogenic shock include simple fainting, spinal cord injury, and the use of anesthetic agents. Therapy should be primarily aimed at restoring and maintaining adequate blood volume by infusing crystalloid solution or by transfusing blood if the patient is anemic. Elevating the legs will help expand the effective blood volume by about 10%. Vascular tone and total peripheral resistance can be increased by the selective use of vasopressor agents that have predominantly α-adrenergic stimulating effects.

▨ Definition

Alterations in vascular resistance can cause hypotension, which may result in the clinical shock syndrome. Neurogenic shock is that clinical shock syndrome that results mainly from a decrease in total peripheral vascular resistance. Like septic shock, neurogenic shock should be classified as a subset of vasogenic shock. Neurogenic shock is a common but rarely fatal cause of shock.

Neurogenic shock is caused by altered vascular resistance. It is a common but rarely fatal cause of shock.

▨ Etiology

There are three main causes of neurogenic shock: 1) neurogenic reflexes producing syncope or fainting, 2) trauma to the spinal cord, and 3) drugs used for spinal, general, or intravenous anesthesia.

Diagnosis

The antecedent history is significant.

The diagnosis of neurogenic shock is usually straightforward. The antecedent history is important. Syncope following pain or the sight of blood or other emotional stimuli usually results from neurogenic reflexes. Other possible etiologies of collapse in this setting include acute myocardial infarction, arrhythmia, and stroke. These must be considered in the differential diagnosis of syncope. A patient who presents with paraplegia or quadriplegia following trauma must be suspected of having a spinal cord injury. The development of hypotension and circulatory insufficiency in this setting must not be assumed to be due to neurologic injury, however, until hemorrhagic or cardiogenic etiologies have been ruled out. Finally, hypotension during anesthesia not attributable to hypovolemia, hypoxia, or coronary insufficiency is most commonly due to the adverse effects of anesthetic agents.

Most patients have warm, dry skin and normal or decreased pulse rate.

The clinical manifestations of neurogenic shock include hypotension, normal or slowed pulse rate, and warm, dry skin. The skin may actually appear flushed. The mental status of the patient in neurogenic shock may range from normal through confusion, lethargy, agitation, stupor, and coma. These alterations are due to changes in cerebral perfusion.

Pathophysiology

There is a mismatch between normal blood volume and vascular capacitance.

The prime pathogenic cause of neurogenic shock is an inhibition of sympathetic vascular tone. This results in a decrease in total peripheral vascular resistance. There is a decrease in the resistance in both the arteriolar resistance vessels and the venous capacitance vessels. Arteriolar resistance decreases as the venous capacitance increases. A mismatch between normal blood volume and overall vascular capacitance occurs. Increased venous capacitance causes pooling of blood in the venous circulation. Ventricular preload will decrease and subsequently so will cardiac output.

In neurogenic shock arteriolar vasodilatation is responsible for the major decrease in peripheral vascular resistance. Venous vasodilation is responsible for the decreased ventricular preload and cardiac output. Obviously, the hemodynamic alterations in neurogenic shock are more pronounced if the patient is hypovolemic prior to shock. If neurogenic shock is not treated, there may result fatal damage to the brain or the heart via cerebral infarction or myocardial infarction, respectively. This is particularly true for the geriatric patient with preexisting cerebrovascular, carotid artery, or coronary artery disease.

> Arteriolar vasodilatation causes a lowered vascular resistance.
>
> Venous vasodilatation causes a lowered cardiac preload.

Fainting is a common cause of neurogenic shock. Certain emotional stimuli (such as pain, loss, etc.) somehow cause the cerebrum to inhibit the cardiovascular center of the medulla. This results in an inhibition of sympathetic nervous activity and an increase in parasympathetic nervous activity. Inhibition of the medullary cardiovascular center causes: 1) a decrease in the resistance of the arteriolar bed, 2) a decrease in the resistance of the venous bed, 3) a decrease in sympathetic cardiac nerve input to the heart, and 4) an increase in parasympathetic cardiac nerve (vagal) input to the heart. This results in a decrease in total peripheral resistance and causes the hypotension of simple fainting.

> The mechanism of fainting

Spinal cord trauma can cause neurogenic shock. Marshall Hall introduced the term spinal shock about 100 years ago. Spinal shock signifies the disappearance of reflex function following anatomic (via blunt or penetrating trauma) or functional (via experimental cold injury) spinal cord section. When the spinal cord is severed, all motor, sensory, and reflex function is abolished below the level of injury. Below the level of injury there occurs paralysis of all muscles, anesthesia of tissues and skin, and abolition of spinal reflexes. There is loss of bladder and rectal function. During spinal shock there is abdominal distention due to ileus, and bowel sounds become hypoactive or absent. Acute intra-abdominal pathology during spinal shock is difficult to identify because of lack of signs of peritoneal or visceral inflammation. Spinal shock occurs within minutes of cord transection and may last several weeks in humans. Gradually spinal reflux function reappears.

> Spinal shock is not equivalent to neurogenic shock.

All sympathetic vaso-
motor control is abol-
ished below the level
of spinal cord injury.

From the above it is clear that spinal shock, which concerns itself primarily with reflex abolition following cord trauma, should not be confused with neurogenic shock complicating cord injury. In addition to the above-described effects of spinal cord transection, there is abolition of all sympathetic vasomotor control below the level of injury. This results in vasodilation of both the arteriolar resistance and the venous capacitance vessels under neural control distal to the site of cord trauma. Total peripheral resistance and cardiac output diminish. This results in hypotension and neurogenic shock.

Anesthesia can cause
neurogenic shock.

Neurogenic shock can also complicate anesthesia. Spinal (subarachnoid) or epidural anesthesia abolishes sympathetic vasomotor control at the level of infiltration. Total peripheral vascular resistance decreases due to vasodilatation of arteriolar resistance vessels and venous capacitance vessels. The overall effect is to produce hypotension.

General (volatile) anesthetics can also cause hypotension and neurogenic shock by inhibiting the vasomotor activity of the medulla. This results in a decrease in sympathetic vasomotor activity. Total peripheral vascular resistance decreases, and venodilation causes a decrease in cardiac preload and output. The result is hypotension. In addition, most general anesthetics can directly depress myocardial contractility. This too will cause a reduction in cardiac output, which contributes to the hypotension.

The cardiovascular ef-
fects of halothane

Halothane is a commonly used general anesthetic. Its cardiovascular effects are several: 1) it decreases sympathetic vasomotor control by medullary inhibition, 2) it directly depresses myocardial contractility, 3) it directly alters the tone of vascular smooth muscle, 4) it blocks the ability of catecholamine (norepinephine) to affect vascular resistance, and 5) it sensitizes the myocardium to catecholamines and thus is arrhythmogenic. The net result is a decrease in total peripheral resistance, cardiac contractility, cardiac output, and blood pressure. Methoxyflurane and enflurane can similarly cause hypotension. Nitrous oxide, however, usually does not cause hypotension. Although nitrous oxide has a minimal depressive effect on myocardial contractility, it also increases the response of vascular smooth muscle to norepinephrine.

During general anesthesia, surgical manipulation can also cause hypotension. Traction on the mesentery, peritoneum, gallbladder, etc., can cause reflex hypotension via parasympathetic (vagal) cardiac nerve fibers. In addition, during surgery there may occur mechanical interference with venous return via the effects of retractors and packs on major veins such as the inferior vena cava.

Surgical manipulation can cause hypotension.

Intravenous anesthetics, such as barbiturates, can on occasion cause neurogenic shock. The cardiovascular effects after the intravenous administration of thiopental, an ultrashort-acting barbiturate, are variable. Some patients respond without any change in mean blood pressure, while others respond with either a decrease or an increase in blood pressure. Ultrashort barbiturates can, however, inhibit the vasomotor activity of the medullary center and depress cardiac contractility by a direct effect. On the other hand, they also have a direct effect on increasing vascular tone. Blood pressure is little affected, since the decrease in cardiac output is accompanied by a usual increase in total peripheral resistance. In barbiturate intoxication, however, hypotension and shock may result from hypoxia, depression of the medullary center, and a direct depressive effect on the myocardium, sympathetic ganglia, and vascular smooth muscle.

Neurogenic shock can be viewed graphically using the systemic and ventricular function curves. In fainting, spinal cord trauma, and spinal anesthesia there is a marked reduction in total peripheral resistance. This reduction in cardiac afterload will tend to rotate the systemic function curve clockwise and shift the ventricular function curve upward and to the left. However, the vasodilation will cause a significant decrease in the effective blood volume and thus cause the systemic function curve to shift downward and to the left (Figure 6.1). This results in a new equilibrium, point C. If general anesthesia is added and myocardial contractility decreases, the ventricular function curve will shift downward and to the right. This results in a new equilibrium, point D, of decreased cardiac performance.

Neurogenic shock can be viewed graphically.

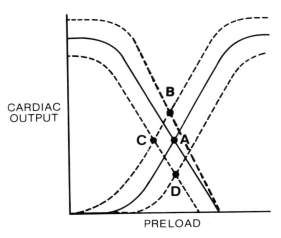

FIGURE 6.1   In neurogenic shock there is initially a reduction in total peripheral vascular resistance. This afterload reduction will cause the systemic function curve to rotate clockwise and the ventricular function to shift upward and to the left. The new equilibrium point B represents improved cardiac performance, but the patient is hypotensive due to the effect of vascular resistance on blood pressure. Simultaneously, there is generalized venodilatation resulting in a decrease in the effective blood volume. This will shift the systemic function curve downward and to the left, resulting in equilibrium point C. If cardiac contractility is then decreased (as in general anesthesia), then the ventricular function curve will shift downward and to the right, resulting in point D.

▬ **Treatment**

The therapy of neurogenic shock involves: 1) removing the causative agent, 2) maintaining adequate blood volume, and 3) the judicious use of vasoactive drugs.

Simple fainting can be treated by placing the patient supine and elevating the legs.

Simple fainting can best be treated by allowing the patient to assume the supine position and by elevating the legs. This maneuver will allow the immediate autotransfusion of about 10% of the total blood volume from the lower extremities to the central great veins. Cardiac preload will be increased, as will cardiac output subsequently. The increased cardiac output will increase blood pressure and will improve cerebral blood flow, thus allowing the regaining of consciousness. If the stimulus for fainting is severe pain or anxiety, this can be alleviated by the administration of analgesics or sedatives, once the patient regains consciousness. The sinus bradycardia that usually accompanies fainting may be treated by an intravenous dose of atropine, 0.5–1.0 mg.

Atropine may be beneficial in treating the sinus bradycardia of fainting.

Neurogenic shock complicating general anesthesia should first be treated by stopping the administration of the causative agent. This is also true for continuous epidural anesthesia. Neurogenic shock caused by spinal cord injury and anesthetic agents can be treated by maintaining an adequate blood volume and by using vasoactive drugs.

Removing the causative agent is important.

The patient's legs should be elevated. As in simple fainting, this will result in an autotransfusion of about 10% of the blood volume and will improve cardiac preload. In neurogenic shock the vascular capacitance is markedly increased due to both vasodilatation and venodilatation. Blood volume can be maintained by the administration of crystalloid solutions, either normal saline or lactated Ringer's. Therapy should begin using boluses of 200–250 ml of these solutions. Hemodynamic responses to fluid therapy should be monitored closely. A CVP or Swan-Ganz catheter is a helpful guide to such fluid therapy. It is important to follow the response in CVP or PCWP to increments of volume loading rather than to concentrate on isolated readings. Once the plateau phase of the ventricular function curve is reached, volume loading should be curtailed so as to avert iatrogenic fluid overload. If the patient is anemic, blood should be used as part of volume therapy.

Volume loading is important. Use crystalloid solutions for this purpose.

A CVP or Swan-Ganz catheter helps to guide fluid therapy.

Most cases of neurogenic shock respond to rapid volume loading. If blood pressure fails to improve following volume loading, then the selective use of vasopressor agents is warranted. Often these agents are used in low doses while volume therapy is being instituted. The goal of therapy is to lessen the mismatch between vascular capacitance and blood volume by fluid therapy and to increase vascular tone and total peripheral resistance by using vasopressors.

Use vasopressor agents cautiously and only when volume loading fails.

Agents that stimulate α-adrenergic vascular receptors and cause vasoconstriction are the drugs of choice since they treat directly the underlying path-ophysiologic abnormality. Several drugs are currently available (Table 6.1). These agents should be administered as a continuous intravenous infusion. The rate of administration depends on the patient's hemodynamic response. Phenylephrine (Neo-Synephrine) is probably the drug of choice for this purpose. It is a potent α-receptor agonist and markedly increases total peripheral resistance. It does so via a direct effect on the α-receptor and also via the release of endogenous norepinephrine. Its pressor effects cause a reflex bradycardia, which can be blocked by the administration of atropine. Cardiac output either remains the same or decreases slightly. The rate of infusion of a solution of phenylephrine (10 mg/500 ml) can be titrated to the individual's hemodynamic response. Methoxamine is a pure α-agonist whose cardiovascular effects are similar to those of phenylephrine. Metaraminol acts as a vasopressor and also increases venous tone. Other drugs that should be considered include mephentermine, ephedrine, and norepinephrine.

Phenylephrine (Neo-Synephrine) is the vasopressor of choice in neurogenic shock.

Case Study

A 20-year-old man falls off a roof while applying new shingles. In the emergency room he is anxious and agitated and complains of some neck discomfort. He is hypotensive with BP 75 mm Hg, pulse rate 90, and respiratory rate 28. On exam there are no signs of trauma, but he is quadriplegic. His neck is stabilized with sandbags. O_2 is given by mask, two large-bore IVs are started in the arms, 2 liters of Ring-

TABLE 6.1   Vasopressor Agents That May Be Used In Neurogenic Shock

Agent	Intravenous Dose
Phenylephrine	10 mg/500 ml
Methoxamine	10 mg/500 ml
Metaraminol	15–100 mg/500 ml
Mephentermine	30 mg/500 ml
Norepinephrine	4 mg/500 ml
Ephedrine	20 mg

Note: Actual rate of infusion of these solutions can be titrated to the patient's hemodynamic response.

er's lactate are rapidly infused, blood work and an ABG are sent, a CVP line is inserted and reads 5 cm H_2O, and a Foley catheter and nasogastric tube are passed. The patient's BP is still only 80 mm Hg after 2 liters of fluid. A peritoneal lavage is performed and is negative. A stat portable lateral C-spine x-ray reveals a fracture-dislocation of C7. Chest x-ray and KUB are negative. Two more liters of Ringer's lactate are infused over the next 15 minutes. BP is now 90 mm Hg and CVP is 10 cm H_2O. Phenylephrine (10 mg/500 ml) infusion is started and BP increases to 110 mm Hg.

The above case illustrates neurogenic shock following spinal cord trauma. Important points to note include: 1) initial stabilization of the neck, 2) fluid resuscitation with crystalloid solution, 3) importance of peritoneal lavage in ruling out significant blunt abdominal injury in causing the hypotension in this setting, and 4) use of an α-agonist vasopressor in increasing vascular resistance and BP after volume therapy. The MAST suit could have been used as well to increase systemic vascular resistance.

Bibliography

Bedbrook G (ed). The Care and Management of Spinal Cord Injuries. Springer-Verlag, New York, 1981.

Dripps RD, Eckenhoff JR, Vandam LD. Introduction to Anesthesia. W. B. Saunders, Philadelphia, 1961.

Prys-Roberts C (ed). The Circulation in Anesthesia. Blackwell, Oxford, 1980.

Ruch TC, Patton HD (eds). Physiology and Biophysics: The Brain and Neural Function. W. B. Saunders, Philadelphia, 1979.

Tibbs PA, Bivins BA, Young AB. The problem of acute abdominal disease during spinal shock. Am Surg pp 366–368, June 1979.

Multiple Organ Failure Syndrome 7

Overview

The multiple organ failure syndrome (MOF syndrome) is that clinical syndrome characterized by failure of multiple organs or biologic systems following any severe metabolic insult such as trauma, shock, surgery, or sepsis. The systems or organs that may fail include the cardiovascular system, the lungs, the kidneys, the liver, the gastrointestinal tract, the metabolic system, the immune system, and the coagulation system. The MOF syndrome usually begins with an episode of circulatory insufficiency accompanied by respiratory failure. The order of organ failure is somewhat variable. Organs begin to fail within 1–2 weeks of injury or operation. Sepsis is the main ingredient in the development of the MOF syndrome. Therapy involves adequate preoperative evaluation, uneventful intraoperative support, and aggressive postoperative management. Prevention and control of infection is the mainstay of effective treatment.

Definition

In the past 10 years it has become evident that many patients dying in surgical intensive care units succumb to failure of multiple organ systems. This is a direct result of our modern ability to sustain critically ill patients with multiple problems. As an example, a patient with mesenteric ischemia may develop the shock syndrome and undergo an urgent operation. Postoperatively the patient develops progressive respiratory insufficiency requiring mechanical ventilatory support. The patient rapidly becomes catabolic. Renal insufficiency and jaundice then develop. The patient appears septic and blood cultures are positive for Gram-negative rods. Upper gastrointestinal hemorrhage from erosive stress gastritis occurs. A coagulopathy may appear. The patient ultimately dies from multiple problems. It is difficult to identify one prime cause of death. This sequence of events has been termed multiple, progressive, or sequential organ systems failure.

The multiple organ failure syndrome (MOF syndrome) is that clinical syndrome characterized by failure of multiple organs or biologic systems following any severe metabolic insult such as trauma, shock, surgery, or sepsis. The systems or organs that may fail include: 1) the cardiovascular system, 2) the lungs, 3) the kidneys, 4) the liver, 5) the gastrointestinal tract, 6) the metabolic systems, 7) the immune system, and 8) the coagulation system.

The MOF syndrome may develop following trauma, shock, surgery, or sepsis.

▩ Etiology

The etiology of the MOF syndrome is complex and only partially understood at present. There are various clinical situations in which the MOF syndrome may develop (Table 7.1). First, there is usually an inciting severe metabolic insult to the patient either from trauma, shock, sepsis, or operation, or some combination of these. An episode of circulatory insufficiency tends to set the stage for the subsequent development of the MOF syndrome. Second, clinical or technical errors may occur which contribute to the development of the MOF syndrome. For example, a bowel anastomosis may be performed under

Clinical situations in which the MOF syndrome may develop

TABLE 7.1   Factors Contributing
to Development of MOF Syndrome

1) Severe metabolic insult:
Trauma
Shock
Surgery
Sepsis
2) Clinical or technical error
3) Infection
4) Preexisting organ dysfunction or disease

excess tension and lead to an anastomotic leak or disruption and cause major intra-abdominal sepsis. Third, infection, either clinically evident or occult, plays a major role in causing the MOF syndrome. Fourth, a patient with preexisting organ dysfunction, such as cirrhosis, diabetes, or obstructive pulmonary disease, would be at increased risk for developing the syndrome.

Polk and colleagues at the University of Louisville found 38 cases of MOF syndrome among 553 patients undergoing emergency operation for both trauma and nontraumatic general surgical emergencies. This represents an incidence of MOF syndrome of about 7% in this patient population thought to be at high risk for the development of the syndrome. The mortality rate of the MOF syndrome was about 75% despite aggressive medical and surgical therapy. The mortality rate increased proportionately to the number of organs failing: one organ 30%, two organs 60%, three organs 85%, and four organs 100% mortality. Various clinical factors were associated with the development of MOF. These included hypovolemic shock, massive volume therapy (blood or crystalloid solutions), chest injury, and sepsis. It should be emphasized that none of these factors were statistically significant in causing the MOF syndrome if the septic patients are omitted.

Sepsis seems to be a necessary ingredient to the subsequent development of the MOF syndrome. The incidence of sepsis in MOF varies between 75% and 100%. The site of infection causing sepsis in this setting is usually intra-abdominal (44–75%) or pulmonary (14–50%).

> Sepsis is a necessary ingredient to the development of the MOF syndrome. The site of infection is usually abdominal or pulmonary.

▨ Diagnosis

The diagnosis of the MOF syndrome can be made once various organs dysfunction or biologic systems fail following trauma, shock, sepsis, or surgery. The MOF syndrome usually begins with an episode of circulatory insufficiency (hemodynamic instability, shock) accompanied by respiratory failure. The patient may be septic from either an intra-abdominal

> The MOF syndrome usually follows an episode of hemodynamic instability.

or a pulmonary source. The order of organ failure is somewhat variable, but usually pulmonary failure is first. Hypoxemia predominates and the patient requires mechanical ventilatory support. Adult respiratory distress syndrome may develop as part of the MOF syndrome. Organs begin to fail within 1–2 weeks of injury or operation.

Hepatic dysfunction causes jaundice. An early initial elevation in total bilirubin level following surgery is usually due to anaesthesia, transfusions, or the absorption of hematoma. The hyperbilirubinemia that occurs as part of the MOF syndrome usually peaks at 8–12 days postsurgery and is usually greater than 2–3 mg%. A persistently elevated bilirubin, however, should indicate an undrained septic focus.

Renal dysfunction may present as either oliguric or nonoliguric acute renal failure. Nonoliguric renal failure usually occurs only in the setting of sepsis. The diagnosis of nonoliguric acute renal failure is made when the urine output remains normal or even supranormal despite rising levels of BUN and creatinine.

Gastrointestinal failure is manifested by bleeding from erosive stress gastritis. Metabolic failure entails a catabolic state. There is depletion of muscle mass, which further interferes with the patient's ability to breathe. The patient loses weight. Immune system failure implies a depressed level of host resistance. Cellular immunity is altered and the patient may become anergic to commonly tested antigens.

The coagulation system too may fail and cause a bleeding disorder. The causes of coagulation system failure include: 1) hepatic dysfunction with depressed production of clotting factors and 2) sepsis. Sepsis, in particular endotoxin, can activate both the coagulation cascade and the fibrinolytic system. This may result in a consumptive coagulopathy typified by thrombocytopenia; an elevation in PT, PTT, and fibrin-split products; and a decrease in fibrinogen titers. The disseminated intravascular coagulation (DIC) syndrome may occur as part of the MOF syndrome.

Hyperbilirubinemia due to the MOF syndrome usually peaks at 8–12 days post-surgery.

Nonoliguric renal failure may occur in sepsis.

Pathophysiology

The pathogenesis of the MOF syndrome is poorly understood at present. As mentioned earlier, this syndrome usually starts with an episode of circulatory insufficiency accompanied by respiratory failure. If the patient is septic or becomes septic following the above events, then the MOF syndrome may develop.

It is known that local or remote infection plays a significant role in the pathogenesis of renal, hepatic, and pulmonary failure following abdominal trauma and surgery. Indeed, failure of these organ systems following trauma, shock, or operation may indicate occult intra-abdominal sepsis. The crucial question of how sepsis causes organs to fail is unresolved. Are there circulatory toxins in sepsis that alter organ function? Is the problem one of local tissue underperfusion, hypoxemia, or altered cellular utilization of oxygen? The answers to these questions remain for future investigational study.

How sepsis causes remote organ failure is unknown.

Treatment

Much has been said about what the MOF syndrome is, which organ or biologic systems it affects, and how sepsis plays an essential role in the syndrome. Until the pathophysiologic details of the syndrome are understood, successful treatment will depend on prevention of the syndrome in the patient at risk and support of organ systems once the syndrome has developed. Using this approach today, physicians are able to salvage only about 25% of these patients. This extremely high and costly mortality rate continues despite aggressive surgical and medical therapy.

Prevention is the key to treatment.

Certain guidelines are available to help prevent the development of the syndrome. In the patient coming to emergent, urgent, or elective major surgery, the preoperative evaluation and intraoperative and postoperative management are all important.

In the emergent situation a detailed preoperative evaluation may be impossible. Under urgent or

Optimizing the patient's medical condition prior to surgery will decrease the postoperative risk of developing the MOF syndrome.

Parameters to evaluate preoperatively

elective situations, however, the patient's overall medical condition should be made optimal prior to surgery (Table 7.2). Pulmonary function and reserve can be measured using formal pulmonary function tests. A bedside measurement of tidal volume and negative inspiratory force may suffice. A baseline room-air arterial blood gas should be obtained. The patient should stop smoking. Breathing exercises and incentive spirometry should be encouraged. The preoperative use of bronchodilators, such as nebulized isoetharine, may be beneficial in improving pulmonary function.

The patient should be evaluated for evidence of cardiovascular disease. This involves physical examination, an EKG, and a chest x-ray. If the patient has evidence of heart failure, digoxin and diuretic therapy should be started preoperatively so as to improve cardiac function. Likewise, identified cardiac arrhythmias should be treated. Renal function can be evaluated by measuring BUN and creatinine levels. If the patient has prerenal azotemia from volume depletion, this should be corrected prior to surgery

TABLE 7.2   Preoperative Assessment and Management

Function	Assessment	Management
Pulmonary	Pulmonary function tests	Stop smoking
	Arterial blood gases	Incentive spirometry
		Breathing exercises
		Bronchodilators
Cardiac	Exam	Digoxin
	EKG	Diuretics
	Chest x-ray	Antiarrhythmics
Renal	BUN	Volume status
	Creatinine	
Liver	Liver function tests	Alimentation
Gastrointestinal system	Peptic ulcer history	Antacids
		Cimetidine
Nutrition	Body weight	Alimentation
	Albumin	
	Transferrin	
Immune competence	Total lymphocyte count	Alimentation
	Skin testing	
Coagulation profile	PT	Vitamin K
	PTT	FFP
	Platelet count	Platelets
Infection	Clinical assessment	Antibiotics
	Cultures	

with judicious intravenous rehydration. Close attention must be paid to electrolyte abnormalities as well.

Anemia should be corrected with transfusion therapy prior to surgery. Hepatic reserve can be measured by obtaining liver function tests. Likewise, a history of alchohol abuse, hepatitis, or cirrhosis should be obtained. The patient should be questioned concerning previous history of peptic ulcer disease, gallbladder disease, pancreatitis, or other gastrointestinal disorders. In a patient with history of prior peptic ulcer the preoperative use of cimetidine or antacids should be considered.

Malnutrition and depressed immune competence are related to increased mortality and morbidity, including the risks of infection and sepsis, following surgery. Ideally, therefore, the patient's nutritional and immune competence status should be evaluated preoperatively, particularly in the high-risk patient. Visceral protein mass can be estimated by measuring serum albumin and transferrin levels. Levels of albumin and transferrin below 3.5 gm% and 200 mg%, respectively, are abnormal. Serum transferrin may serve as a more accurate assessment of protein malnutrition, since its half-life (8–10 days) is shorter than that of albumin (20 days). Thus transferrin levels will be depleted earlier in protein malnutrition than will albumin levels.

How to evaluate for immune competence and malnutrition

Immune competence can be estimated by the total lymphocyte count, which is calculated by multiplying the white blood cell count by the percentage of lymphocytes present on differential count and dividing by 100. A total lymphocyte count below 2000 per mm^3 is abnormal, and a level below 800 per mm^3 indicates severe depletion. Alternatively, cell-mediated immunity can be tested using skin test antigens such as tuberculin, *Candida*, *Trichophyton*, mumps, and streptokinase-streptodornase. An anergic response indicates depressed host resistance.

Preoperative nutritional support with either enteral supplements or peripheral or central hyperalimentation may restore immunocompetence and improve wound healing. Surprisingly, clinical trials are still needed to prove the efficacy of preoperative nutritional support in preventing postoperative sepsis and decreasing overall surgical morbidity and mortality.

Preoperative nutritional support may be indicated.

Coagulation abnormalities should be corrected.

It is important also to check a coagulation profile (PT, PTT, and platelet count) preoperatively. An elevated PT may indicate underlying hepatic insufficiency. Clotting factors can be restored by giving fresh frozen plasma. Occasionally a hereditary clotting factor deficiency may be identified. Platelets should be made available if the thrombocyte count is below 50,000 per mm^3.

Prophylactic antibiotics may be indicated, and antibiotics should be started during the critical period of bacterial invasion, within 4 hours of injury.

Prophylactic antibiotics, usually a cephalosporin, should be used in certain circumstances, particularly in cardiovascular procedures. With tissue injury, such as abdominal trauma or compound fracture, antibiotics should be started during the critical period of bacterial invasion. This is usually within 4 hours of injury. Thus, in trauma surgery antibiotics should be started in the preoperative phase of treatment in order to be optimally successful in the prevention of wound infection or sepsis.

Intraoperative management is also important (Table 7.3). The anesthesiologist and the surgeon must work in concert. The dose of volatile inhalation anesthetic must not be excessive.

Maintain organ function during surgery.

Organ function must be maintained during surgery. This involves aggressive monitoring of blood pressure, pulse, urine output, blood loss, arterial blood gases, and sometimes cardiac output. Technical surgical errors should be avoided at all cost.

Postoperative circulatory support may require volume therapy, inotropic agents, vasopressors, or unloading agents.

Postoperative care involves several areas of support (Table 7.4). Circulatory support involves maintaining normovolemia. This may require blood or crystalloid infusion if the patient is hypovolemic. A central venous pressure or Swan-Ganz catheter should be used to guide volume therapy. The Swan-Ganz catheter can also be used to measure cardiac output. Inotropic support with dopamine, dobutamine, digoxin, epinephrine, or isoproterenol may become necessary. Sometimes it is necessary to lower ventricular afterload in order to improve cardiac performance. Sodium nitroprusside or occasionally an intra-aortic balloon pump can be used for this pur-

---

TABLE 7.3   Intraoperative Caveats

1) Avoid toxic anesthetic dose
2) Maintain organ function with aggressive monitoring
3) Avoid technical errors

TABLE 7.4   Postoperative Assessment and Management

Function	Assessment	Management
Pulmonary	Arterial blood gases	Volume respirators
	Chest x-ray	PEEP
	Pulmonary capillary wedge pressure	Diuretics
		Avoid albumin
Cardiac	Blood pressure	Normovolemia
	Pulse	Inotropic drugs
	Urine output	Vasopressors
	Central venous pressure	Afterload reduction
	Pulmonary capillary wedge pressure	
	Cardiac output	
Renal	Urine output	Normovolemia
	BUN	Maintain cardiac output
	Creatinine	Diuretics
	Urine sodium	Dialysis
Liver	Liver function tests	Maintain cardiac output
		Nutritional support
Gastrointestinal	Nasogastric tube	Nasogastric tube
	Gastric pH	Antacids
		Cimetidine
Nutrition	Albumin	Enteral feedings
	Transferrin	Peripheral hyperalimentation
	Body weight	Central hyperalimentation
		Vitamins
		Trace elements
		Intralipid
Immune competence	Total lymphocyte count	Nutrition
	Skin testing	
Coagulation system	PT	Vitamin K
	PTT	FFP
	Platelet count	Platelets
Infection	High index of suspicion	Antibiotics
	Cultures	Drain septic foci
		Consider reexploration

pose. Sometimes a vasopressor agent, such as norepinephrine or phenylephrine, is needed.

Ventilatory support should be used early and liberally, particularly in patients at high risk of pulmonary failure such as those with preexisting obstructive lung disease and peritonitis. The alveoli should be kept well expanded using a volume respirator, intermittent mandatory ventilation, and positive airway pressure. Pulmonary toilet using endotracheal suctioning should be frequent. If there is fluid overload, diuretics should be used to decrease interstitial pulmonary edema and improve oxygenation. Albumin therapy in most cases should be

Ventilatory support should be used early.

avoided, since it may increase interstitial pulmonary fluid and contribute to pulmonary insufficiency.

Renal function may be preserved by maintaining normovolemia and cardiac output. Diuretics or dialysis, if needed, should be used early. A patient in high-output renal failure from sepsis may be hypovolemic despite good urine volumes. A urine sodium of less than 20 mEq/liter is a clue to this situation. This patient would require volume therapy so as to prevent the further insult of hypovolemia on renal function.

In high-output renal failure avoid hypovolemia.

The jaundice of hepatic insufficiency in the MOF syndrome is usually due to a hypoxemic insult and cholestasis. Treatment is usually nonspecific and includes nutritional support and maintenance of hepatic blood flow. Other causes must be ruled out, such as hepatitis, biliary infections, or intra-abdominal sepsis.

Gastrointestinal hemorrhage from stress gastritis should be prevented. A nasogastric tube should be passed and placed on low suction. Antacids (30–120 ml/h) with or without cimetidine (300 mg q4–6h) can be used to titrate gastric pH above 4 and toward 7.

Use antacids liberally.

Nutritional support should start early so as to prevent or correct malnutrition and to maintain immune competence. The gastrointestinal tract should be used if functional. At surgery it may be wise in the high-risk patient to insert a feeding jejunostomy catheter for this purpose. Central total parenteral nutrition may be necessary. Intralipid infusion should be used both as a noncarbohydrate calorie source and to prevent essential fatty acid deficiency. Vitamins and trace elements should also be administered.

Nutritional support is necessary.

Finally, it is most important to prevent and control infection. Antibiotics should be started preoperatively with tissue injury and within 4 hours of contamination. All areas of septic foci must be drained and removed. This includes not only intra-abdominal abscesses but also infected vascular catheters (peripheral or central lines) and infected Foley catheters. Abscesses must be drained. In peritonitis the abdomen may be irrigated with bacitracin or a cephalosporin solution to afford some increased antimicrobial action.

Surgery may be necessary to control infection.

As stated earlier, pulmonary, hepatic, or renal insufficiency following trauma or surgery may indicate occult intra-abdominal infection. When organ failure occurs in the postoperative patient, a high index of suspicion of occult intra-abdominal abscess should be maintained. This is true even if a non-invasive work-up (including gallium scans, ultrasound, and CT scan) is nondiagnostic. These patients should be strongly considered for reexploration.

Annotated Bibliography

Baue AE. Multiple organ or system failure. In: Haimovici H (ed), Vascular Emergencies. Appleton-Century-Crofts, New York, 1981.
A detailed review of this syndrome.

Baue AE, Chaudry IH. Prevention of multiple systems failure. Surg Clin North Am 60:1167–1178, 1980.
A discussion of the prevention of multiple organ failure syndrome.

Eiseman B, Beart R, Norton L. Multiple organ failure. Surg Gynecol Obstet 144:323–326, 1977.
A clinical study of this syndrome.

Fry DE, Pearlstein L, Fulton RL, et al. Multiple system organ failure. Arch Surg 115:136–140, 1980.
A comprehensive clinical study on the cause and treatment of multiple system organ failure.

Polk HC Jr, Shields CL. Remote organ failure: A valid sign of occult intra-abdominal infection. Surgery 81:310–313, 1977.
Clinical evidence is presented to support the fact that remote organ failure can occur as a result of intra-abdominal infection.

Additional Bibliography

Baue AE. Multiple, progressive or sequential systems failure. Arch Surg 110:779–781, 1975.
Baue AE. Sequential or multiple system failure. In: Najarian JS, Delaney JP (eds), Critical Surgical Care.

Symposia Specialists Medical Books, Miami, pp 293–300, 1977.

Border JR, Chenier R. McMenamy RH, et al. Multiple systems organ failure: Muscle fuel deficit with visceral protein malnutrition. Surg Clin North Am 61:437–463, 1976.

MacLean LD. Host resistance in surgical patients. J Trauma 19:297–304, 1979.

Tilney WL, Bailey GL, Morgan AP. Sequential system failure after rupture of abdominal aortic aneurysms. Ann Surg 178:117–122, 1973.

Index